THE COST OF BIRTH DEFECTS

Estimates of the Value of Prevention

Norman J. Waitzman
Richard M. Scheffler
Patrick S. Romano

University Press of America, Inc.
Lanham • New York • London

Library of Congress Cataloging-in-Publication Data

Waitzman, Norman
The cost of birth defects : estimates of the value of prevention /
Norman J. Waitzman, Richard M. Scheffler, Patrick S. Romano.
p.   cm.
Includes index.
1. Abnormalities, Human--Costs. I. Scheffler, Richard M. II.
Romano, Patrick S. III. Title.
RG627.W294   1994   362.1'95043--dc20   95-50912 CIP

ISBN 0-7618-0247-9 (cloth: alk. ppr.)
ISBN 0-7618-0248-7 (ppr: alk. ppr.)

Contents

List of Tables

v

Preface

Birth defects have now surpassed both prematurity and sudden infant death syndrome as the leading cause of infant mortality in the United States. Most infants with birth defects, however, do not die in infancy. Depending on the birth defect and the affected individual, considerable medical treatment may be administered throughout adulthood. For several defects that are not fully correctable through early medical treatment, functional and activity limitations often ensue that require additional services for developmental support, special education, and rehabilitation. These limitations may hinder performance in the household and the workplace where, consequently, productivity losses also may be substantial. As evidenced by recent legislation, such as the Americans with Disabilities Act, society is responding with renewed sensitivity to the growing voice of the disabled and their advocates for expanded access at school, work, and other social institutions. As the costs associated with enforcement of such access increase, so does the relative value of prevention of disability. This book lays the groundwork for appraising such value and weighing different policy options with respect to birth defects.

Despite the substantial personal and societal effects related to birth defects and their treatment, a surprisingly limited amount of research has attempted to measure the economic costs of birth defects in the aggregate or individually. The research that has been performed to date has mostly been limited in scope or method. This book represents a major effort to fill these gaps with respect to eighteen of the most clinically significant birth defects that affect approximately 35,000 newborns each year in the United States. We have combined newly generated incidence and mortality data from the California Birth Defects Monitoring Program with data on medical treatment, special education services, developmental services, activity limitations, and earnings to generate the most comprehensive estimates to date on the societal costs of these conditions.

The results of our analysis suggest that, in aggregate, these eighteen birth defects alone have an annual national cost of more than $8 billion (in 1992 dollars). This aggregate estimate is indicative of the important societal significance of this particular category of illness. However, birth defects also are diverse in terms of their underlying pathogenesis and their effects on health and function. The estimates of cost for individual defects from our analysis provide the basis for allocating research funds and appraising prevention strategies. Indeed, our detailed assessment of a folate supplementation program to prevent neural tube defects, drawing on our cost estimates for spina bifida, is provided in the final chapter. Depending on the level of folate supplementation, our analysis suggests that such a program would generate benefits that are 3.3 to 4.6 times greater than the costs.

The cost-of-illness analysis presented in this book is unusual in its union of medical and economic expertise. All too often in cost-of-illness studies critical aspects of the disease process are seriously compromised by data limitations or the exigencies of method. We have, therefore, taken extra care to place medical expertise on an equal footing with economic theory by integrating insights from expert researchers and clinicians into our methodology and by bringing to bear an impressive array of new data to the subject. Health economists and health services researchers, those in the medical community who have an interest in congenital anomalies and their treatment, and policymakers and other stakeholders in the health policy arena will have a special interest in this book.

Health economists and health services researchers will quickly discover that this book is tantamount to a hands-on primer on cost-of-illness methodology. General economic and philosophical principles and assumptions underlying cost-of-illness methodology are reviewed, and the book also is painstaking in its detail of how to perform a cost-of-illness study. A step-by-step description of the method (with respect to each category of cost) and how actual data (with all of its limitations) can be adapted to the methodology are contained in the book. The presentation, while specific to birth defects, is provided on a level in which there can be general application to specific, common problems encountered in cost-of-illness studies. This "how-to" character of the book, we believe, will be of service to those in the fields of applied health services research and teaching.

Health services researchers will be attracted, as well, by several refinements that we have incorporated into standard cost-of-illness methodology and the accessible exposition concerning such refinements. We based our medical cost estimates on financial records of medical utilization specific to each disease rather than relying on average cost of visits and stays across disease categories, as is often the case in the cost-of-illness literature. The complex issues surrounding the cost of comorbidities are treated with greater sensitivity in this study than in studies that routinely attribute costs solely to a primary diagnosis. We did not assume that each unit of service in which the disease is reported as a contributing diagnosis adds to incremental cost, but instead constructed total cost profiles of those with the disease and subtracted that of the average person so as to better approximate the true incremental cost of each illness. Whereas cost-of-illness investigators often estimate the value of lost productivity due to illness strictly on the basis of an estimate of lost workdays, we made innovative adjustments to account for potential reductions in wages as well.

Cost-of-illness studies increasingly have branched into the important area of nonmedical direct costs, incorporating estimates of such costs as rehabilitation and special education services. We have extended these efforts in our analysis by constructing estimates of nonmedical direct costs that are based on actual records of placement and treatment related to each condition rather than adopting gross averages from the available literature.

The medical community should take interest in the lifetime profiles of individual diseases presented in this book. Population estimates that are presented related to receipt of treatment and services and to functional limitations in school and work related to individual conditions may be somewhat surprising in particular instances in light of strict clinical experience. The incidence approach undertaken in the analysis places an emphasis on the potential societal savings through prevention. Stakeholders in the policy arena will take particular interest in the estimates of the relative costs of individual conditions and the profile of services presented in this book in weighing competing strategies for treatment and prevention.

Chapter 1 provides a general overview of the overall importance of assessing the societal impact of birth defects, particularly given the paucity of prior research. Summary estimates of costs are presented. In three sections, Chapter 2 covers both general and specific methodological issues in the application of cost-of-illness methodology to birth defects. The first section maps out our resolution of general methodological issues. The second summarizes how a two-dimensional classification of birth defects was relevant for estimating costs. The final section is devoted to the development of a more specific methodology, and the general equations developed there are used throughout the remainder of the book. In Chapter 3, population estimates (incidence, prevalence, and survival) that are used throughout the study are presented. Chapter 4 presents our method for estimating direct medical costs and provides our final estimates of such costs. Chapter 5 is devoted to two categories of nonmedical direct cost estimates: developmental services and special education. We provide our estimates of indirect costs of birth defects in Chapter 6. In Chapter 7, we provide summary cost estimates for both California and the nation. These estimates also are discussed in the context of earlier cost-of-illness literature with respect to birth defects. Our detailed cost-benefit analysis of a program of folate supplementation of food to prevent neural tube defects also is presented in Chapter 7, based partially on our findings with respect to the cost of spina bifida. This first-of-its-kind analysis demonstrates that the benefits of such a program exceed the costs by a large margin. Finally, we present evidence on the research effort devoted to birth defects in the United States.

Acknowledgments

The authors would like to thank all of those who graciously gave their time and expertise and contributed to the successful completion of this book.

We are grateful to the members of our medical advisory panel for their contributions: Lucy S. Crain, MD, MPH, Department of Pediatrics, University of California, San Francisco; Philip H. Cogen, MD, PhD, Department of Neurological Surgery, University of California, San Francisco; Robert E. Piecuch, MD, Department of Pediatrics, University of California, San Francisco; Michael Heymann, MD, Cardiovascular Research Institute, University of California, San Francisco; N. Scott Adzick, Department of Surgery, University of California, San Francisco; and Stephen R. Skinner, MD, Shriner's Hospital for Crippled Children, San Francisco.

We would like to thank our panel of economic advisors for their insights regarding methodology and for comments on earlier drafts: Dorothy P. Rice ScD (Hon), Institute for Health and Aging, University of California, San Francisco; Teh-wei Hu, PhD, School of Public Health, University of California, Berkeley; and Ciaran Phibbs, PhD, Center for Health Care Evaluation, Veterans Administration Medical Center, Menlo Park, California.

We also are appreciative of the comments given by Jeffrey Gould, PhD, School of Public Health, University of California, Berkeley; John A. Harris, MD, MPH, Chief, California Birth Defects Monitoring Program; Paul Newachek, PhD, Institute for Health

Policy Studies, University of California, San Francisco; and Joy Grossman, PhD.

This study benefitted from the expert programming assistance provided by Konstantinos Tsatsaronis, Harish Chand, Barney Cohen, and Lasse Bergman.

Several research assistants contributed to the compilation of relevant literature and data. In this regard, we would like to acknowledge the contributions of Marshall Schiff, Sande Okelo, Anne White, Elliott Marseille, Eleanor Bried, Randy Pi, and Stephanie Bender-Kitz.

In the California Department of Developmental Services, we would like to extend a special thanks to James White for generating the special data set from the Department used in this study and for graciously meeting with us and lending his expertise with respect to the Department's activities. Other public officials in several departments deserve our recognition. Although we ultimately do not report results from data acquired from the California Children Services Branch of the California Department of Health Services, we are grateful for the efforts of Donn Johnson, Chief of the Administrative Support Section, for providing California Children Services data. We also would like to thank Robert Barnhouse in the Department of Health Services for his programming support in this regard. Similarly, data from the California Department of Rehabilitation were graciously provided by Takao Iwasa, Chief of the Statistics Section. Several individuals in the California Department of Education were instrumental in providing data regarding special education services and in helping us understand the delivery of these services in California and the nation. These include Dawn Casteel, Bill Fong, Dale E. Badgley, and Lalit M. Roy.

For their secretarial and word processing support, we are indebted to Joan Chamberlain, Hildegarde Wilson, Pat Gatton, and Carolyn Bennion.

Finally, we would like to express our gratitude to the California Birth Defects Monitoring Program and the March of Dimes for their financial support, without which this book would not have been possible.

Chapter 1

Introduction

Birth defects are the leading cause of infant mortality in the United States, surpassing both prematurity and sudden infant death syndrome. The percentage of infant deaths attributable to birth defects has increased from 7% in 1916-1919 to 20.5% in 1986.[1] These deaths account for approximately 5.4% of all years of potential life lost before age 65. Most children with birth defects, however, do not die in infancy. Depending on the defect and its severity, special medical treatment may be required into adulthood. Medical care is often not fully corrective, making birth defects a major cause of childhood and adult disability as well. In addition to medical services, significant societal resources including special education, rehabilitation, and other nonmedical services are devoted to treat those born with congenital anomalies. Productivity is lost because of premature mortality and heightened morbidity.

The importance of preventing congenital anomalies recently has received increased focus in national health policy. In *Healthy People 2000*, the Public Health Service's report of national objectives for health promotion and disease prevention, reduction of and better knowledge regarding congenital anomalies are highlighted as requirements for reducing infant mortality in the country.[2] In *Beyond Rhetoric*, the final report of the National Commission on Children, which included then-Governor Bill Clinton as a commissioner, birth defects are cited as major contributors to the chronic and disabling conditions affecting 10% to 15% of children in the United States that require renewed attention through public policy.[3]

Despite the considerable societal and personal impact of birth defects and the increasing political commitment to child health and welfare, little is known about the economic burden to society of birth defects or the costs of certain defects relative to others. In the latest of a series of aggregate analyses of the cost of illness in the United States, congenital anomalies, as a group, were estimated to cost $6.3 billion in 1980, or 1.4% of the total cost of illness.[4] This estimate included direct medical care costs and productivity loss due to premature mortality. Nonmedical direct costs such as special education and developmental services, were not incorporated. Productivity losses due to heightened morbidity in adulthood from these conditions were found to be of minor significance. It is likely that such morbidity costs and other costs were underestimated because all costs were attributed to a single, primary diagnosis, whereas birth defects may often be an important factor in the development of, and add significantly to the cost of, coexisting illnesses. Furthermore, data limitations in this aggregate analysis were likely responsible for underestimating mortality and morbidity costs associated with birth defects. The highly aggregate nature of the study also steered it toward relying much more on average costs for categories of services rather than the actual costs of services provided for certain illnesses. Inpatient hospital costs, for example, were based on the average cost of an inpatient day multiplied by an estimate of the number of inpatient days related to the illness. Outpatient visits to the hospital and doctor were treated in a similar fashion. This methodology, of course, ignores the variation of intensity of stays and visits related to particular diseases.

To date, few estimates have been made of the costs of individual birth defects, although some studies have focused on the costs and benefits related to prenatal screening for neural tube defects[5,6,7] and for Down syndrome.[8,9,10] Most of these studies were conducted on populations outside of the United States, several used data that are now outdated, and few generated comprehensive estimates of direct and indirect costs that have become standard in the cost-of-illness literature. A recent study on the cost of brain disorders estimated the direct and indirect costs of cerebral palsy to be $1.2 billion in 1991 based on a methodology similar to the aggregate study by Rice et al. above.[11] Costs of long-term care in institutional facilities and special education were not incorporated.

We estimated the cost of eighteen of the most clinically significant birth defects in the United States using an incidence approach from standard cost-of-illness methodology. Under this approach, we estimated the indirect mortality and morbidity costs and direct costs of medical, developmental, and special education services over the entire life span of those born with each defect in California in 1988.

Our summary estimates of the societal cost of each individual defect projected to the nation, as well as the aggregate cost of all eighteen conditions, are provided in Table 1-1. The aggregate costs for these conditions ranged between $3.2 billion and $19.5 billion, depending on the discount rate applied to costs after the first year of life. Using a middle, 5% discount rate as a best estimate, the aggregate cost for the nation in 1992 was $8 billion. Even though not directly comparable to the aggregate estimates cited above, these estimates suggest that the cost of birth defects significantly exceeds those estimates when adjustments are made for better comparison.[a,12] The cost of specific defects also were sensitive to the discount rate; but the cost for conditions associated with relatively high incidence, coupled with substantial activity limitations over the life span such as spina bifida, cerebral palsy, and Down syndrome, tended to have the highest overall costs and large costs per case regardless of the rate of discount selected.

The summary breakdown of estimates at a 5% discount rate by cost category is given in Table 1-2. Each direct and indirect cost category contributed significantly to the overall $8 billion in cost. Indirect costs summarize lost productivity from premature mortality and heightened morbidity. These costs ($5 billion) comprised more than 60% of total aggregate costs, whereas direct medical, special education, and developmental services comprised the other 40%. Medical costs comprised approximately one-quarter of total aggregate costs and two-thirds of total direct costs.

The heterogeneity of the conditions partly is reflected in the wide range in the relative size of specific direct and indirect cost categories across conditions (Table 1-2). Heart conditions have very high medical costs, as well as high costs related to infant mortality. The

---

[a]A direct comparison of our estimates to those in the aggregate analysis by Rice et al. after performing several adjustments is provided in Chapter 7.

Table 1-1. Summary costs of birth defects, United States ($1,000s, 1992)

Condition	Total cost by discount rate			Cost per case by discount rate		
	2%	5%	10%	2%	5%	10%
Spina bifida	1,035,284	489,289	237,602	622	294	143
Truncus arteriosus	420,982	209,676	121,390	1,015	505	292
Transposition/DORV	1,208,636	514,529	233,235	625	267	121
Tetralogy of Fallot	715,617	360,486	207,535	521	262	151
Single ventricle	415,355	172,631	71,644	827	344	143
Cleft lip or palate	1,852,051	696,501	229,285	267	101	33
TE fistula	370,383	165,002	83,221	325	145	73
Atresia, small intestine	203,233	110,061	72,234	138	75	49
Colorectal atresia	542,776	219,262	90,736	305	123	52
Renal agenesis	1,222,794	424,159	111,351	720	250	65
Urinary obstruction	938,347	343,223	110,035	230	84	27
Upper-limb reduction	442,720	170,036	56,856	257	99	33
Lower-limb reduction	452,156	167,067	50,457	537	199	60
Diaphragmatic hernia	963,890	364,348	128,185	663	250	89
Gastroschisis	217,440	108,763	65,305	217	108	65
Omphalocele	338,682	132,004	50,294	452	176	67
Down syndrome	4,560,483	1,847,752	700,064	1,113	451	171
Cerebral palsy	5,771,954	2,425,781	926,833	1,196	503	192
Total cost	19,546,742	8,030,672	3,170,933	N/A	N/A	N/A

Note: Figures are based on lifetime direct and indirect cost estimates for the 1988 birth cohort in California adjusted for differences in births and costs between California and the nation, as well as for cost inflation between 1988 and 1992. Costs beyond the first year of life were discounted back to the year of birth at the rate indicated. Column totals are less than column sums because total cost estimates reflect a downward adjustment in order to avoid double counting due to multiple conditions of interest. See Chapter 7 for greater detail on the methodology for computing summary totals.

Table 1-2. The cost of birth defects in the United States, by cost category, discounted at 5% ($1,000s, 1992)

Condition	Direct costs			Indirect costs (c)	Total costs
	Medical (a)	Special education (b)	Developmental services (b)		
Spina bifida	204,512	41,672	1,781	241,324	489,289
Truncus arteriosus	107,578	602	--	101,496	209,676
Transposition/DORV	166,334	4,402	--	343,794	514,529
Tetralogy of Fallot	185,122	3,974	--	171,390	360,486
Single ventricle	61,659	871	--	110,101	172,631
Cleft lip or palate	97,126	17,551	2,937	578,888	696,501
TE fistula	61,558	--	--	103,444	165,002
Atresia, small intestine	63,156	--	--	46,905	110,061
Colorectal atresia	57,213	--	--	162,049	219,262
Renal agenesis	24,713	--	--	399,466	424,159
Urinary obstruction	46,294	--	--	296,929	343,223
Upper-limb reduction	11,138	24,280	--	134,619	170,036
Lower-limb reduction	16,560	11,851	--	138,656	167,067
Diaphragmatic hernia	62,772	--	--	301,576	364,348
Gastroschisis	54,520	--	--	54,243	108,763
Omphalocele	27,871	--	--	104,133	132,004
Down syndrome	278,696	293,960	95,029	1,180,068	1,847,752
Cerebral palsy	851,809	226,718	217,899	1,129,355	2,425,781
Total cost	2,104,419	591,842	295,557	5,038,854	8,030,672

Note: Figures are based on lifetime direct and indirect cost estimates for the 1988 birth cohort in California adjusted for differences in births and costs between California and the nation, as well as for cost inflation between 1988 and 1992. Costs beyond the first year of life were discounted back to the year of birth at a 5% discount rate, a rate commonly used in cost-of-illness studies. Column totals are less than column sums because total cost estimates reflect a downward adjustment in order to avoid double counting due to multiple conditions of interest. See Chapter 7 for greater detail on the methodology for computing summary totals. Row totals may not equal row sums because of rounding.

(a) Estimates of medical care costs are for care through the second year of life for conditions listed in quadrant I of Table 2-2 with the exception of colorectal atresia, for which estimates are through age seventeen. Congenital urinary tract obstruction may be associated with medical costs beyond the second year, but data limitations prevented estimation of such costs. For conditions listed in other quadrants of Table 2-2, estimates reflect costs through age sixty-five.

Table 1-2. (Continued)

(b) Estimates are provided only for conditions for which there was an expectation of above-average rates of disability (those listed in quadrants II and IV of Table 2-2). Data limitations prevented us from estimating developmental and special education services costs associated with renal agenesis and developmental services costs associated with heart anomalies and limb reductions.

(c) Indirect costs reflect lost productivity because of excess mortality and morbidity. The mortality cost component includes costs associated with excess first-year mortality for all birth defects except for three listed in quadrant IV of Table 2-2: (a) spina bifida (through age nine), (b) Down syndrome (through age sixty-five), and (c) cerebral palsy (through age seventeen). Even though excess mortality beyond the first year is likely for other conditions listed in that quadrant, data limitations prevented us from making such estimates. The morbidity cost component was estimated only for conditions listed in quadrants II and IV of Table 2-2. Data limitations prevented us from estimating morbidity costs associated with renal agenesis.

direct costs for special education for children with Down syndrome, on the other hand, exceed the direct costs of medical services for individuals born with that condition.

Nearly one of every seven births in the United States occurs in California, and the state houses the California Birth Defects Monitoring Program (CBDMP), one of the most extensive active surveillance efforts with respect to birth defects in the world. We combined newly generated prevalence and survival data from the CBDMP with resource utilization, work and school limitation, and cost and earnings data from several sources under a unified methodology to generate estimates that are the most comprehensive to date.

A summary of the eleven major data sources that we used for our estimates, how birth defects were identified from these sources, and the way we utilized each source in estimating cost are provided in Table 1-3. In Appendix 2, we provide a brief, but fuller, description of each of these data sources.

Our estimates provide the basis for comparisons across birth defect categories and establish the necessary groundwork for assessing prevention strategies in cost-benefit and cost-effectiveness analyses. In the final chapter, we present an economic analysis with respect to a program of folate supplementation of food to prevent spina bifida and anencephaly based on our total cost estimates. We found that the benefits of such a program are significantly greater than the costs, even under the most restrictive assumptions.

Basic research is the first stage toward development of this and any other future birth defect prevention program. The fiscal crisis facing the nation makes such basic research, in which the return is, by its very nature, uncertain and sometimes seemingly remote, an easy target for budget cuts. Squelching public funds for research for lack of immediate returns, however, poses the danger of short-sightedness with respect to the types of cost-saving opportunities presented by the proposed folate program above.

Decisions also must be made over allocation of the societal research budget, regardless of its size and the extent to which it is growing or shrinking. It should be kept in mind, however, that cost-of-illness methodology captures that which we can quantify–generally in monetary terms, possibly at the expense of other, less easily quantifiable, societal values. The intent of our analysis is to inform more fully the public debate over how to allocate best our public and private resources with respect to health care and research and to lay the groundwork for future studies of economic cost that build on our estimates.

Table 1-3. Summary of major data sources used to estimate the costs of birth defects (a)

Data source	Years	Sample	Birth defect identification	Usage in population estimates	Usage in cost estimates
CBDMP1—California Birth Defects Monitoring Program incidence data	1983-1988, pooled	All California births in ascertainment area (b)	BPA codes (c)	Incidence (I) (e) Prevalence, ages zero to one (PREVPOP)	
CBDMP2—California Birth Defects Monitoring Program linked birth death records	1983-1986, pooled	CBDMP1 linked to death records	BPA codes (c)	Survival, ages zero to one (m)	
NHIS—National Health Interview Survey	1985-1989, pooled	US noninstitutionalized population	ICD-9 recodes	Prevalence, ages two plus (PREVPOP) Proportions requiring special education, limited in work (p)	
OSHPD—California Office of Statewide Health Planning and Development hospital discharge abstracts	1988	All discharges from California acute-care, nonfederal hospitals	ICD-9-CM codes		Medical inpatient, outpatient
MediCal—MediCal "tape-to-tape" claims file	1988	All California claims reimbursed by MediCal	ICD-9-CM codes		Medical inpatient, outpatient, long-term care
DDS—California Department of Development Services (DDS) master file	1988-1989, fiscal year	10% of those in California receiving DDS services	ICD-9 codes	Proportions requiring developmental services, long-term care (f) (p)	Developmental services
SRI—The National Longitudinal Study of Special Education Students	1985	US population receiving special education services	Condition list/handicap category (d)	Distribution among handicap category (fc)	

Table 1-3. (Continued)

Data source	Years	Sample	Birth defect identification	Usage in population estimates	Usage in cost estimates
SEED—California Special Education Enrollment Data	1988-1989, school year	California school district enrollment data	Handicap/placement category	Distribution of California students by category (CALPROP)	Special education
SPEND—California Special Education Expenditure Data	1988-1989, fiscal year	California school district expenditure data	Handicap/placement category		Special education
SIPP—Survey of Income and Program Participation, Wave 2	1987	US noninstitutionalized population	Disability status/condition list		Morbidity
CASEP—California Age-Sex Earnings Profiles	1989	US earnings adjusted to California	None		Mortality/morbidity

(a) A brief description of these data sources is provided in Appendix 2.

(b) The CBDMPI ascertainment area progressively expanded over the period to cover nearly all counties in California by 1988.

(c) British Pediatric Association (BPA) codes are very similar to International Classification of Disease, 9th edition (ICD) codes but allow for greater specificity.

(d) The mapping of conditions to federal handicap category on SRI permitted the linkage to SPEED and SPEND based on federal handicap category.

(e) Incidence data on cerebral palsy were not available from CBDMPI (Chapter 3).

(f) Estimates from DDS of the proportion requiring long-term care in state development centers were made only for those with Down syndrome and cerebral palsy.

Endnotes to Chapter 1

1.Centers for Disease Control. Contribution of birth defects to infant mortality—United States. *Morbidity and Mortality Weekly Report.* 1989a;38:633-635.

2.US Department of Health and Human Services, Public Health Service. *Healthy People 2000: National Health Promotion and Disease Prevention Objectives.* DHHS Publication No. (PHS) 91-50212. Washington, DC: US Government Printing Office; 1991.

3.US National Commission on Children. *Beyond Rhetoric: A New American Agenda for Children and Families.* Washington, DC: Author; 1991.

4.Rice DP, Hodgson TA, Kopstein AN. The economic costs of illness: a replication and update. *Health Care Financing Review.* 1985;7(1):61-80.

5.Hagard S, Carter F, Milne RG. Screening for spina bifida cystica: a cost-benefit analysis. *Br J Prev Soc Med.* 1976;30:40-53.

6.Centers for Disease Control. Economic burden of spina bifida—United States, 1980-1990. *Morbidity and Morality Weekly Report.* 1989b;38:264-267.

7.Tosi LL, et al. When does mass screening for open neural tube defects in low-risk pregnancies result in cost savings? *CMAJ.* 1987;136:255-263.

8.Glass N. Economic aspects of the prevention of Down's syndrome (mongolism). In: Bailey NTJ and Thompson M., eds. *Systems Aspects of Health Planning.* North-Holland Publishing Co.; 1975.

9.Hagard S, et al. Ibid.

10.Mikkelsen M, Nielsen G. Cost-benefit analysis of prevention of Down's syndrome. In: Boue, A. ed. *Prenatal Diagnosis.* Paris: Les Colloques de L'Institut National de la Recherche Medicale. 1976;61:283-289.

11.National Foundation for Brain Research. *The Cost of Disorders of the Brain.* Washington, DC: Author; 1992.

12.Rice DP, et al. Ibid.

Chapter 2

The Application of Cost-of-Illness Methodology To Birth Defects

The methodology associated with estimating the cost of illness rests on both economic principles and philosophical assumptions regarding pathogenesis and the nature of cost. This chapter is divided into three sections. The first section is devoted to general issues in cost-of-illness methodology that are relevant to estimating the cost of birth defects. We make explicit some of the important underlying principles and assumptions in cost-of-illness methodology and explain the manner in which we addressed critical methodological issues and incorporated refinements into our application. The second section is devoted to a brief discussion of the nature of birth defects and a general typology that was developed for estimating their costs. The third section provides a more specific model of cost estimation given the general methodological approach and typology for birth defects. The general or basic equations developed there provide the basis for discussing the computation of estimates of each cost component in subsequent chapters.

The Resolution of General Methodological Issues

Evolution of Cost-of-Illness Methodology

The pioneering cost-of-illness studies in the late 1950s and early 1960s[1,2,3,4] addressed the distinction between direct and indirect cost under what has come to be known as the human capital or "livelihood" approach. Under this approach, earnings are viewed as returns to education, medical care, and other resources with an "investment-like" character. Direct cost includes all resources used or "invested" to treat illness and disability such as medical care and developmental services. Indirect cost includes all resources lost to society from reduced productivity due to premature mortality and heightened morbidity. Under the human capital approach, estimates of cost are based on market valuations of used and lost resources as opposed to individual valuations of a reduction in risk of experiencing an adverse event such as a birth defect. The latter approach, based on principles of welfare economics, has been described as "willingness to pay" and usually leads to higher estimates of the value of life.[5] Some of the relative strengths and weaknesses of the two approaches are described below.

Applications of cost-of-illness methodology have evolved over time from focusing on the cost of very broad disease categories to examining more specific diseases so that the relative benefits of competing treatment and prevention strategies can be assessed. An early emphasis on medical costs also has given way to greater emphasis on other types of direct services such as special education and rehabilitation, that may add substantially to the cost of illness.[6,7,8]

In our application, we were sensitive to these extensions. In addition to direct medical cost, we estimated the direct cost of developmental and special education resources devoted to children and adults with birth defects. Furthermore, we focused on eighteen separate birth defects, and our methodology, as described below, was sensitive to differences among them.

Direct and Indirect Costs

Two types of costs generally are estimated under standard cost-of-illness methodology: (a) direct costs and (b) indirect costs. Direct costs are costs associated with resources *used* to treat and support people with underlying conditions of interest. Indirect costs are resources *lost* to society such as lost productivity, because of premature mortality and heightened morbidity associated with illness.

In addition to estimates of traditional "core" direct costs related to medical care (inpatient, outpatient, long-term care, appliances, pharmaceuticals, and lab tests), cost-of-illness has progressively branched out in recent applications in making estimates of other types of direct costs. Other direct costs include resources used for developmental services and special education for those with chronic disabilities.

People born with several of the birth defects that we analyzed have higher rates of activity limitations as children and adults than do those in the general population. We, therefore, made estimates of the direct cost associated with developmental services and special education devoted to support people with birth defects that lead to activity limitations.

Society loses the productivity of those who die or become limited in their ability to work due to illness, and this indirect cost can be estimated based upon lost expected earnings. Such foregone earnings in cost-of-illness studies are usually estimated based upon cross-sectional labor force participation and earnings profiles by age and sex in the general population. A profile of total earnings is relevant for estimating the loss to society due to premature mortality or limitations that render a person completely unable to work.

For those who are limited in the amount or type of work, however, an estimate must be made of the reduction in lifetime earnings due to such limitations. It has been customary in the cost-of-illness literature to estimate such reductions based strictly on restricted activity days (reductions in the amount of work only) and assume that wage rates for those with limitations are the same as in the general population. In the current study, we incorporated adjustments for differences in earnings and labor force participation in addition to the amount of work in estimating this "amount or type" component of indirect costs of birth defects due to morbidity (Chapter 6).

Resources lost to society (indirect cost) include lost household production, as well as lost labor market earnings. Estimates of lost household production by age and sex based upon an analysis of household tasks and the market price for performing such tasks are incorporated in cost-of-illness studies, including the current study, to generate more comprehensive figures on indirect cost (Chapter 6).

Even though indirect costs due to the devotion of parents or other family members' time for caretaking of children with birth defects also are appropriate to incorporate in cost-of-illness methodology, we did not make such "noncore," indirect cost estimates in our study. In this respect, our estimates of indirect costs are conservative.

The Human Capital Approach

The concept of direct cost may seem less abstract than indirect cost in the sense that the resources devoted to care and support of those with birth defects are already-produced, palpable goods and services, whereas indirect costs involve never-produced goods and services. The same counterfactual regarding the absence of illness and the resulting deployment or redeployment of resources, however, undergird both categories of cost. In the absence of birth defects, resources currently invested to support and treat those with illness would be freed up to invest elsewhere. Similarly, in the absence of illness, human resources would be less impaired and, therefore, more productive.

The "investment" character of direct and indirect cost, as described above, characterizes what has come to be known as the "human capital" approach. From an economic perspective, the stream of lifetime earnings represents a return to direct investments in education, training, medical care, and other forms of "human capital." Direct costs of medical care, developmental services, and special education, in other words, are seen as investments in human capital. Indirect cost represents the value to society of the lost return to such investments.

Some theorists have questioned the "investment" character of these expenditures, however, because the return in increased labor market productivity resulting from them is often unlikely to exceed the "investment."[9] Instead, these resources are likely expended by individuals, families, and private and public organizations to improve the overall quality of life and to preserve the dignity of those with birth defects based on ethical principles. Lipscomb, therefore, forwards an expanded view of human capital investment to include increases in "consumption efficiency" (the enjoyment of life of those with birth defects) rather than to focus exclusively on efficiency in production. This perspective preserves the investment orientation to the theoretical underpinning of cost-of-illness methodology. Lipscomb terms this expanded view the "livelihood approach." Under this approach, the cost to society from birth defects is the net resources devoted to and foregone for those born with birth defects relative to children born without birth defects. The "net" aspect of this calculation is discussed further below.

In contrast to the societal "investment" focus of the human capital approach, the willingness-to-pay approach attempts to assess the cost of illness on the basis of what individuals or society would pay to reduce the probability or risk of its occurrence. This approach represents an attempt to be comprehensive in incorporating all subjective valuations, such as pain and suffering, in addition to the value of tangible resources invested. It is more closely aligned with the concept of "opportunity cost" in economic theory. However, attempts to operationalize this approach and to assess what individuals or society are willing to pay in the absence of overt markets that provide such information often falter in the use of surveys or surrogate markets that provide incomplete or unreliable information.[10]

Because willingness-to-pay estimates are generally higher than human capital estimates, many have come to regard human capital estimates as minimum cost estimates. Similarly, in arguing for a broader "livelihood" concept of investment, it was noted above that private and public expenditures on medical care, developmental services, and special education for those who have severe disabilities are hardly "rational investments" in the traditional sense of expectation regarding greater future returns. Outside of a strict investment framework, these expenditures can be viewed alternatively as "net" expenditures that individuals and society are willing to pay to promote an acceptable minimum quality of life for individuals with birth defects. Given such willingness, one might presume that society would be willing to pay this level at minimum for prevention.

The Relevant Population: Incidence Versus Prevalence

An important issue for any cost-of-illness study is the relevant population for making cost estimates. Until recently, most studies, consisting of the aggregate cost-of-illness study that included an estimate for all congenital anomalies,[11] have estimated costs for the prevalent population (a cross-section of the population with the disease of interest at a given time). More recent studies have estimated the lifetime profile of costs for the incident population, that is, those newly diagnosed with an illness during a calendar year.[12,13,14] Data requirements for the incidence approach are usually more formidable because per-person costs at each stage of the illness must be estimated. Practical considerations such as ease with which population and cost data can be acquired can, therefore, dictate which approach is adopted in cost-of-illness studies. From a theoretical standpoint, however, the two approaches have come to be associated with different emphases on prevention versus treatment.

The prevalence approach is considered to be more appropriate for assessing treatment strategies, whereas the incidence approach is better suited to the assessment of prevention strategies.[15] The cost per incident case is the potential benefit of each case prevented.

Our underlying interest in laying the groundwork for assessment of birth defect prevention strategies steered us toward adopting an incidence approach. The costs that we estimate are, therefore, costs over the life span for those born with birth defects of interest in the base year: 1988. The cost of interventions that reduce the number of incident cases can be compared directly to the reduction in costs or, equivalently, the level of benefits from such interventions in formal cost-benefit analysis. One such analysis of folate supplementation of grains to prevent neural tube defects such as spina bifida is provided in the final chapter.

Associated Anomalies and Incremental Costs

We made cost estimates for individuals with birth defects rather than the costs of the birth defects per se. Birth defects often are associated with other conditions such as low birthweight; thus, it would be very difficult to disentangle from total costs the costs exclusively to the condition of study. Also, the treatment of the person rather than the condition as the unit of analysis fits well with the emphasis on prevention under the incidence approach. Presumably, if the birth defect is prevented, associated anomalies also would be prevented. Of course, conditions that are not associated with the underlying condition would not be prevented and should not be included in cost estimates of the disease. We, therefore, attempted to isolate only the incremental cost related to the condition of interest and associated anomalies, as described in more detail below.

The treatment of comorbidities in cost-of-illness studies actually reflects underlying assumptions about the disease process or pathogenesis. If certain disease processes are completely independent of the condition under study, then it would be inappropriate to include the costs of such independent comorbidities as a cost of the illness of interest. A certain percentage of those with cerebral palsy, for example, also have mental retardation. If the underlying pathogenesis of mental retardation is totally independent of that of cerebral palsy, then it would be inappropriate to include the costs associated with mental retardation as a cost of cerebral palsy for a person who has both conditions.[a] On the other hand, the fact that cerebral palsy surfaces in a certain portion of the population in its pure form without mental retardation is not necessarily an indication that the two are fully independent. As Koopman and Weed[16] have maintained, there may be several underlying causes and pathways leading to a particular disease. Some pathways may produce various combinations of comorbidities, whereas others may lead to disease without comorbidities. Unfortunately, as discussed further below, pathogenesis in the area of birth defects is rarely known with certainty. If one process leading to cerebral palsy invariably involves the development of mental retardation, then the complete prevention of cerebral palsy also would prevent mental retardation along this pathway, and the costs of mental retardation appropriately would be included as a cost of cerebral palsy in such cases.

---

[a]Of course, even if the underlying causes of the two conditions were completely independent, the treatment of one could be affected by the existence of the other. Costs associated strictly with treatment for mental retardation, in other words, may be higher than average because cerebral palsy adds complications to such treatment. On the other hand, if there are common facets of treatment for both conditions, then the existence of cerebral palsy may reduce the marginal cost of having mental retardation.

Disease processes are such that the presence of a single risk factor is not necessarily sufficient for a particular disease to develop, however.[17]   Certain underlying causes of cerebral palsy, in other words, may act as a risk factor for mental retardation, but mental retardation may develop only if other component risk factors also are present. The underlying pathogenesis for cerebral palsy would be partially responsible only for such instances of mental retardation. In fact, these cases of mental retardation presumably could be prevented without preventing cerebral palsy if other component factors necessary to the development of mental retardation in the presence of cerebral palsy were prevented. The possibility of shared and unshared risk factors suggests the existence of intermediate associations between the poles of total independence and full dependence among comorbidities. The basis for attribution of cost in the event of such intermediate processes is less straightforward than in either of the extreme cases.

It also is worthwhile to note that our interest in laying the groundwork for assessment of prevention rather than treatment strategies is important to the manner in which comorbidities are regarded and handled in our cost-of-illness study. If, in the above example, the treatment of cerebral palsy has no effect on mental retardation, then a cost of cerebral palsy study aimed at assessment of treatment strategies might justifiably ignore the cost of mental retardation, even if its underlying pathogenesis was connected to cerebral palsy.

Cost-of-illness researchers often do not make sufficiently explicit these complications of cost attribution related to underlying pathogenesis. The methods by which costs are tabulated in all cost-of-illness studies, however, contain at least an implicit subscription to an underlying disease process that may or may not correspond to the process that is present.   In order to circumvent the potential problems of comorbidities, for example, costs are oftentimes tabulated strictly from records of episodes of treatment for which the condition of interest is listed as the primary condition. In this manner, the episode of care is treated as the unit of analysis, and each unit is allocated exclusively to one disease. This method is adopted in the aggregate analysis by Rice et al.,[18] as well as a recent study on the cost of brain disorders.[19]   The implicit theory of pathogenesis in such studies is that of "independent disease processes."   Rice and Kelman' s[20] analysis of the incremental hospital costs of alcohol, drug abuse, and mental illness as comorbidities addresses some of the problems in this area and incorporates crude adjustments when alcohol, drug abuse, and mental illness disorders are listed as a secondary diagnosis. Even though the assumption of independent disease processes may appear to be a conservative methodology, it is one that will distribute costs incorrectly if other types of pathogenic processes are at work. Costs related to underlying causes that seem remote or secondary to the most immediate or primary cause will be underestimated, whereas costs related to the primary cause may be exaggerated. Furthermore, the cost of disease as an aggregate of episodes of care also ignores the fact that some modified form of care may have taken place absent the primary diagnosis.[b,21]   In the case of delivery by caesarean section because of a particular complication of pregnancy, for example, the appropriate baseline to estimate incremental costs might be normal delivery rather than no care.

   Other cost-of-illness studies that also have used the episode of care as the unit of analysis have figured cost by summing all such episodes for which the diagnosis of interest was recorded as the primary or as any secondary diagnosis. This method assumes a pathogenic process of strict dependence and may lead to overestimation of cost for a single diagnosis. A cost-of-epilepsy study using this method, for example, has been criticized for attributing to epilepsy costs that are more appropriately attributable to other causes.[22]   In studies that make cost estimates for more than one disease, this methodology also has the drawback of preventing direct aggregation across disease categories without double-counting episodes of care that have more than one of the diagnoses of interest listed.

   We attempted to capture intermediate disease processes in our methodology by focusing on all costs for the person with a disease of interest, whether or not the diagnosis happened to appear on the record of a specific episode of care. We decided to subtract the costs for the average person in order to identify actual incremental costs related to the disease. Low birthweight in any specific instance may or may not be an associated anomaly of a birth defect, for example. Because it occurs among births in which no birth defect is present, low birthweight also is part of a disease process that is independent

---

[b]This point also was made in the cost of brain disorders study (endnote 19).

of that for any particular birth defect. In subtracting the average cost among the general population from the cost among those with birth defects, we attempted to subtract such independent processes and isolate the incremental cost associated with diseases in intermediate and dependent processes. We, therefore, subtracted "average" direct and indirect costs in our estimates in order to generate the "incremental" cost associated with birth defects. More detail on how we accomplished such net calculations for each of the cost components is described in the respective component cost chapters and sections of the book.

This method of estimating incremental costs has the potential limitation of attributing costs to diseases that are more appropriately attributable to prior or higher-level disease processes. The sequential or hierarchical nature of the disease process, in other words, is an additional factor in pathogenesis that is of import. In the hypothetical example above with respect to cerebral palsy as a risk component for mental retardation, cerebral palsy was assumed to be causally prior to mental retardation. If we were to perform a cost study of mental retardation and included the cost of cerebral palsy for those who had both mental retardation and cerebral palsy, we would tend to overestimate the cost of mental retardation because the disease might be prevented without having any impact on cerebral palsy through the elimination of component risks for mental retardation other than cerebral palsy. On the other hand, the prevention of cerebral palsy would prevent a certain number of cases of mental retardation, that is, those for which all component factors necessary for the development of mental retardation were present except those related to cerebral palsy.

Similarly, those born with Down syndrome have a higher risk of cleft deformity than among the general population. If the pathogenic process is such that one would have to prevent Down syndrome in order to prevent this associated deformity, then the cost of Down syndrome among those with both defects is incorporated appropriately as a cost of the cleft deformity. However, if Down syndrome is only one risk component in a disease process leading to a cleft deformity that requires the presence of other risk factors as well, then the inclusion of the total cost of Down syndrome in the cost of cleft deformities for those with both defects, under our methodology, overstates the cost of the cleft deformity. In such a case, the cleft deformity associated with Down syndrome may be preventable through the eradication of these other risk factors. The fact that most of the defects we analyzed are major structural defects, all of which are manifest at birth, suggests that these conditions are likely at a high level along any pathogenic process that results in associated anomalies and that the above problem generally would be minor. Furthermore, the absence of a full longitudinal profile of treatment on individuals with birth defects made it unlikely that we were able to capture all services provided to such individuals. The subtraction of generally reliable average costs of services from what are likely underestimates of total consumption of such services among those with conditions of interest also tended to bias our estimates of incremental costs downward. The discussion in Chapter 4 of our adjustment of inpatient costs, based on hospital discharge abstract data using MediCal (California' s Medicaid program) claims data that have a longitudinal component, provides some insight into the nature and scope of this problem.

Because of associated anomalies, our cost estimates by condition are not directly additive across birth defect categories. Infants born with Down syndrome, for example, also have a greater than average chance of having a congenital heart defect as well. Some of the same people are, therefore, included in our cost estimates for Down syndrome as in our cost estimates for heart conditions. Adding the two cost categories together would, therefore, entail double counting. Data from the CBDMP, however, indicated that the extent of this overlap was relatively small. Approximately 90% of those born with the defects we analyzed did not have any of the other defects. As described in Chapter 7, we made an aggregate cost estimate by developing an algorithm that allocates cost for those with multiple defects to a single defect category based on the CBDMP data.

Incremental Over What? An Underlying Counterfactual

In cost-of-illness studies, there is an implicit counterfactual, that is, what would have occurred absent the disease or intervention being analyzed. Cost should be measured against such a baseline. This counterfactual is not always the same but instead reflects the underlying purpose and structure of the study. For example, some studies have undertaken a cost-benefit analysis of a program of prenatal screening for neural tube defects such as spina bifida.[23,24] A certain percentage of those screened likely would terminate the pregnancy and then proceed to attempt and conceive what is termed a "replacement" child. The appropriate baseline against which the costs of spina bifida is measured in such studies is, therefore, that of the replacement child. Because our analysis focuses on complete prevention, however, pregnancies presumably would culminate in births absent such defects. Costs would revert to that of an "average" person. We, therefore, estimated incremental costs based upon the birth of an "average child" in place of the child with birth defects.

Requirements Versus Effective Demand

Our estimates of cost are based on effective demand, that is, actual patterns of utilization of services and labor market participation and earnings. In this sense, our cost estimates are based on what actually transpired rather than an independent medical or otherwise normative assessment of what was required or would have been optimal. Perhaps some infants born with congenital anomalies such as spina bifida do not receive optimal medical care because they are not adequately covered by insurance or otherwise face barriers to access. Perhaps lower labor force participation and earnings among those with Down syndrome reflects, to a certain degree, labor market discrimination rather than lack of skills. Our estimates of costs do not reflect ideal conditions, that is, optimal treatments and potential earnings under conditions of perfect competition, but conditions as they exist. These costs are the likely savings through immediate prevention strategies. Of course, with changes in policy that bring the actual state of affairs closer to the ideal, cost estimates would change.

Discounting of Future Costs

Under economic theory, current consumption is valued over future consumption. A dollar at present is, therefore, more valuable than a dollar in the future. This tenet underlies the economic theory of real interest on savings. Costs that are incurred in the future, therefore, must be discounted in order to be expressed in terms of present value. The further into the future costs are incurred, the more heavily such costs are discounted to reflect present value.

The concept of present discounted value is easily illustrated by an example of interest on savings. If $100 is placed into a savings account today at a simple annual interest rate of 10%, there will be $110 in the account after a year, $100 multiplied by $(1+.10)$. In the second year, one would have $121, which is $110 multiplied by $(1+.10)$, or $100 multiplied by $(1+.10)^2$. This example can be generalized to the formula of future value (FV): $FV = PV*(1+i)^r$, where PV is the present value ($100), i is the rate of interest (.10), and r is number of years over which interest accrues.

Conversely, $110 a year from now (or $121 two years from now) has a present value of $100 assuming the same 10% rate of interest. A simple manipulation of the above formula generates the formula for present value of future costs or returns: $PV = FV/(1+i)^r$.

Because we estimated direct and indirect costs over the life span for those born with birth defects in 1988, cost estimates were generated for future years. In order to express all cost estimates in terms of present value, we accordingly discounted estimated future costs to the present. The timing of costs over the life cycle is, therefore, a major factor in terms of the impact of discounting on costs. Because all of the incident cases in our study were newborns by definition, all future costs were discounted to birth. For costs incurred to treat birth defects early in life such as a major proportion of medical care for several of the defects, r was low and the effect of discounting was, therefore, small. For costs generally incurred in adulthood, however, the dampening impact of discounting on costs (r) was particularly large. Because earnings are typically concentrated in later years, for example, indirect costs due to birth defects were reduced considerably by the convention of discounting.

Aside from the timing of costs, the size of the discount rate (i) is the other major factor in the effect of discounting on costs. The higher the discount rate (i), everything else equal, the lower the present value of future costs. Even though economists agrce in principle on the concept of discounting future costs, there is not widespread agreement on the "correct" discount rate. Several rates are generated in security markets, depending on risk and other factors. Furthermore, security markets reflect the aggregate of individual valuations, whereas cost-of-illness attempts to estimate societal valuations. If society has a longer time horizon over which it invests than individuals, then the relevant discount rate may be lower than that generated in securities markets.

Cost-of-illness studies often provide a range of estimates based on different discount rates and then provide summary estimates based upon a middle rate such as 3%, 4%, or 5%. We accepted this convention in our calculation of the cost of birth defects and provide cost estimates at 2%, 5%, and 10%. Some detailed estimates are provided at a 5% discount rate, which is common in the cost-of-illness literature.

A Typology of Birth Defects Relevant To Estimation of Costs

Birth Defect Categories

Birth defects are heterogeneous in terms of their underlying pathology and their effects on health and functioning. Even though there are more than 200 different types of birth defects,[25] we chose to analyze eighteen, listed with their corresponding International Classification of Diseases, 9th Revision (ICD-9) codes in Table 2-1, on the basis of their clinical significance and broad spectrum of organ system involvement. Although cerebral palsy is not generally considered a birth defect, we treated it as such because it is defined as a static encephalopathy with motor manifestations that originate during the perinatal period.

Two dimensions of these birth defects related to the usual course of illness were particularly relevant to estimating their costs: postinfancy survival probability and long-term disability. Prior to elaborating on these two important dimensions, we provide a brief, general overview of what little is known regarding the pathogenesis of birth defects, which illustrates their heterogeneous nature and effects.

The Causes of Birth Defects

Despite the social, economic, and emotional impact of birth defects, as well as their substantial cost to society, the causes of birth defects and the mechanisms by which they develop are poorly understood. Many environmental agents that cause abnormalities of development in the human fetus, called teratogens, have been identified. Nonetheless, research to determine how these teratogens induce abnormal development have been complicated by several factors.

Table 2-1. Birth defect categories for which cost estimates were made

Organ system	Condition	ICD-9/BPA codes (a)
Central nervous system	Spina bifida	741.0x, 741.9x
Heart	Truncus arteriosus	745.0
	Transposition/DORV	745.1x
	Tetralogy of Fallot	745.2
	Single ventricle	745.3
Gastrointestinal	Cleft lip or palate	749.0x, 749.1x, 749.2x
	TE fistula	750.3
	Atresia, small intestine	751.1
	Colorectal atresia	751.2
Genitourinary	Renal agenesis	753.0
	Urinary obstruction	753.2
Musculoskeletal	Upper-limb reduction	755.2
	Lower-limb reduction	755.3
	Diaphragmatic hernia	756.6
	Gastroschisis	756.7
	Omphalocele	553.1
Syndromes	Down syndrome	758.0
Other	Cerebral palsy	343.x

Note: See Appendix 1 for a description of each birth defect.

(a) British Pediatric Association (BPA) codes are identical to all but three of the listed ICD-9 (International Classification of Diseases, 9th edition) codes except that BPA codes allow for greater specificity (extra digits). BPA codes for transposition/DORV and for gastroschisis differ slightly from ICD-9 codes with respect to the fifth digit. The BPA code for omphalocele is 756.70x.

Most birth defects occur as a consequence of not one but several related factors, and their interrelationship can be complex or obscure. Few ideal models of birth defects in animals extrapolate to the human condition.   Individuals vary in their susceptibility to teratogens.   Interactions among different agents[26] and random

variation in the occurrence of rare events (such as the birth of a child
with a particular defect) confound research in teratogenesis. The
pitfalls of epidemiologic studies (such as the difficulties faced in
selecting participants and in obtaining unbiased accounts of maternal
exposures to potential teratogens) make defining the causes of birth
defects an even more daunting task.

Despite these difficulties, substantial progress has been made in
finding the causes of birth defects. Known infectious teratogens
include rubella virus (which causes German measles),
cytomegalovirus, varicella-zoster virus (which causes chickenpox),[27]
and syphilis. High-energy radiation, fever,[28] and sauna or hot tub
exposure[29] may be physical teratogens.   Ethyl alcohol,[30]
warfarin,[31] cocaine,[32,33] thalidomide,[34] noncontraceptive steroid
hormones,[35] and anticonvulsants such as phenytoin[36] and
carbamazepine[37] have all been implicated as chemical teratogens.
Studies of occupational differences in the risk of birth defects suggest
that chemical solvents,[38] paints,[39] and pesticides[40] also may be
teratogenic. Mothers who have hyperglycemia caused by diabetes
mellitus are markedly more likely than others to have a child with
congenital anomalies.[41,42]   Several clinical trials involving women
with a prior history of a fetus or child with a neural tube defect
suggest that folic acid deficiency may increase the risk of recurrence
in subsequent pregnancies.[43,44,45,46]   Despite these findings, only
approximately 20% of all birth defects can be attributed to a
teratogenic exposure. Known genetic factors, often exposed by
inbreeding, account for a similarly small proportion of birth
defects.[47,48]   The risk of birth defects other than chromosomal
abnormalities is probably not related to the mother' s age.[49]

Congenital anomalies are abnormalities present when a child is
born. They may be hereditary or they may be caused by a factor that
influences development during the child' s gestation in the womb. In
either case, they take many varied forms. Some are relatively minor
cosmetic problems, whereas others are universally fatal. Some
serious anomalies are completely correctable, whereas others are
chronic conditions that confer lifelong disability. Some anomalies
occur as solitary defects, whereas others are often part of a complex
of associated anomalies. Some result from an adverse influence on
fetal development occurring within four weeks after conception,
whereas others may originate during labor and delivery. Most birth
defects are apparent at birth or shortly thereafter, but some are not

evident at birth and remain undiagnosed until early adulthood or even until after the individual dies a normal death.

Treatments — Because the effects of birth defects are so varied, the treatments offered to affected children also vary substantially. If a birth defect involves a structural abnormality, the most important aspect of treatment is often surgery to correct the disorder. Most congenital defects of the heart, diaphragm, palate, and gastrointestinal tract, for example, can be repaired. The surgery may be complex, however, and it may require several operations over many years to achieve a satisfactory result. Surgical correction typically is performed as soon as the child' s condition allows; that is, the earlier in the child' s life such procedures are performed, the better are healing and physiological function. Timely operations are particularly important for infants with congenital heart disease; that is, they may develop irreversible pulmonary hypertension (high blood pressure in the lungs), leading to congestive heart failure, if surgical repair is unduly delayed. The major exception to this principle is for defects that are not life threatening but that cause stable functional impairments such as cleft lip or palate and orthopedic anomalies like extra fingers or webbing between fingers or toes. For those birth defects, surgical correction is usually delayed until impairment of the child' s ability to function becomes noticeable or until the child is old enough to participate in therapy and rehabilitation.

For many defects, surgical correction is only one aspect of a multidisciplinary treatment program. Prolonged rehabilitation may be necessary to gain optimal functional ability, especially for children with orthopedic defects. Braces or appliances help affected children to participate in school and recreational activities, but occupational and physical therapy are often essential. Correction of certain gastrointestinal defects may reduce the amount of digestive tract available for absorbing nutrients, and, in such cases, nutrition becomes a long-term concern. Children with spina bifida have abnormalities of their bowel and bladder function that require a lifelong program of self-catheterization and medical therapy in order to maintain urinary continence. Speech therapy may be necessary for children undergoing the surgical correction of cleft lip, cleft palate, or both.

Another group of birth defects cannot be resolved or improved with any type of surgical intervention. These defects involve several organs or body systems, or they involve physiological impairments not related to any defect of anatomic structures. Chromosomal abnormalities such as Down syndrome (trisomy 21) and trisomy 18 are classic examples of this group. Genetic diseases such as cystic fibrosis and Huntington' s chorea also may fall into this category, but those disorders are not within the scope of this study.

For this study, we selected a group of birth defects that are neither comprehensive nor representative but that include at least one of the serious defects that affect each major organ system. Following are ten of the major birth defects that occur most frequently: spina bifida, conotruncal heart anomalies, cleft deformities of the lip or palate, tracheoesophageal fistulas, intestinal atresia or stenosis, kidney or urinary tract malformations, congenital limb reductions, congenital diaphragmatic hernia, abdominal wall defects, Down syndrome, and cerebral palsy. These ten defects are divided into eighteen clinically distinguishable subtypes (Table 2-1), which are individually described in more detail in Appendix 1.

Common dimensions relevant to cost—Two dimensions of birth defects related to the usual course of illness were particularly relevant to estimating their costs: postinfancy survival probability and long-term disability. These dimensions are presented as the axes of the 2x2 matrix in Table 2-2. Defects listed in quadrant I of Table 2-2 tend to be characterized by an acute phase at birth that often requires medical attention through infancy. First-year survival among infants born with these defects generally is dependent on the success of early surgical correction and medical care. The likelihood of normal life span and functioning among first-year survivors is very good, suggesting that the subsequent cost of illness is low. For this group of defects, we, therefore, concentrated on direct medical costs through the second year of life and indirect mortality costs through the first year of life.[c] Colorectal atresia was an exception in the limited sense that we expected additional medical care to be potentially required through age seventeen. Because long-term

---

[c]Urinary tract obstruction may be associated with additional medical care after the second year if the diagnosis is established late. However, our analysis focused exclusively on cases diagnosed during infancy. The two-year cutoff for estimating direct medical costs was selected to capture the cost of routine postoperative care.

Table 2-2.   Classification of birth defects by survival and disability status

| | | Postinfancy disability rates among survivors | |
		Average	Above average
		(I)	(II)
	Normal	TE fistula	Cleft lip or palate
		Atresia, small intestine	Upper-limb reduction
		Colorectal atresia	Lower-limb reduction
		Urinary obstruction	
Survival		Diaphragmatic hernia	
after first		Gastroschisis	
year		Omphalocele	
		(III)	(IV)
	Below normal	[None]	Spina bifida
			Truncus arteriosus (a)
			Transposition/DORV (a)
			Tetralogy of Fallot (a)
			Single ventricle (a)
			Renal agenesis (a)
			Down syndrome
			Cerebral palsy

(a) The clinical literature suggests that most congenital heart defects and renal agenesis or dysgenesis are probably associated with excess mortality beyond the first year of life. Unfortunately, there are no population-based studies of long-term survival among children with these anomalies in the modern era. In addition, our estimates of first-year mortality from CBDMP2 were significantly higher than the levels reported in surgical case series. We, therefore, took a conservative stance and assumed normal survival beyond the first year.

disability is unusual with all of these defects, nonmedical direct costs and indirect morbidity costs were assumed to be relatively unimportant.

Those born with defects listed in quadrant II of Table 2-2 also were treated as experiencing elevated mortality only through the first year of life. However, medical care for these defects may not be fully corrective and often extends well beyond the second year. Nonmedical direct costs (such as those related to developmental services and special education) are likely to be significant as well. Indirect morbidity costs must be considered because some people with these conditions suffer disabilities that persist into adulthood.

Those born with spina bifida, congenital heart anomalies, renal agenesis, dysgenesis, Down syndrome, or cerebral palsy (quadrant IV of Table 2-2) also often have lifelong disabilities that require both continued medical attention and other direct services.   Indirect morbidity costs are likely to be significant as well. These conditions differ from those in quadrant II, however, in that excess mortality continues throughout life. Our indirect mortality costs for those born with spina bifida, Down syndrome, and cerebral palsy reflect this extended period of decreased survival. Unfortunately, we could not estimate indirect mortality costs beyond the first year of life for cardiac anomalies, renal agenesis, or dysgenesis because there is so little recent literature describing the long-term survival of these patients.[d,50,51,52] Data limitations also prevented us from estimating nonmedical direct costs and indirect morbidity costs associated with renal agenesis or dysgenesis.

Basic Formulas for Estimating Costs Under the Incidence Approach

A General Formulation for the Cost of Birth Defects

Under the incidence approach that we adopted, direct and indirect costs were estimated for the entire life span of the cohort born with congenital anomalies in the base year, that is, the newly "incident" cases in 1988. A general formulation for our cost estimates is provided in Equation 2-1:

$$COBD = \Sigma_i TC_i / (1+r)^i, \hspace{2cm} [2\text{-}1]$$

where the cost of each birth defect (COBD) is equal to the sum of total incremental costs (TC) over the life span for the cohort born with the defect in 1988. Costs incurred beyond the base year (the year of birth) are discounted at the rate, r, back to the base year. The index, i, therefore, also happens to equal the average age of the cohort (in years).

In this general formulation, TC represents the sum of component incremental direct and indirect costs ($\Sigma_j TC_j$). Direct costs are attributable to medical care, special education, and developmental services. Indirect costs are attributable to lost productivity from

---

[d]Now that most cardiac anomalies are surgically repaired in infancy, late mortality is probably 10% or less.

premature mortality or heightened morbidity. The general
methodology we adopted for estimating these j direct and indirect
component parts of incremental total cost (TC) is outlined below.

A General Formula for Total Cost

Under the incidence approach, one would ideally gather a true
longitudinal profile of direct and indirect costs over the lifetimes of
those born with congenital anomalies in the base year. This is
impossible, of course, given that our base year was 1988 and much of
the relevant resource utilization and productivity losses will occur in
the future as the 1988 cohort ages. Instead, we estimated the
longitudinal profile of resource utilization and lost productivity for
each defect based on recent cross-sectional data on the prevalent
population. Per-capita-cost estimates by age group from such cross-
sectional data multiplied by estimates of the size of the incident
cohort at each age yielded total age-specific cost estimates for the
incident cohort. Equation 2-2 summarizes this methodology:

$$TC_{ij} = (S_i) \times (PCPREV_{ij}),\qquad\qquad [2\text{-}2]$$

where TC_{ij} is the total incremental cost of a particular j set of
services provided (e.g., medical care or special education) to or lost
(productivity) from the incident cohort at age i; S_i is an estimate of
the number alive in the incident cohort at age i;* and $PCPREV_{ij}$ is
the per-capita cost of such resources among affected individuals at
age i.

Per-capita costs in the prevalent population, $PCPREV_{ij}$, are equal
to the ratio of total costs in the prevalent population ($TCPREV_{ij}$)
divided by the size of that population ($PREVPOP_i$). Equation 2-2
can, therefore, be rewritten:

$$TC_{ij} = (S_i) \times (TCPREV_{ij}/PREVPOP_i).\qquad\qquad [2\text{-}3]$$

In order to illustrate this methodology, suppose that children born
with a particular birth defect experience above-average medical costs

---

*In the case of indirect costs from premature mortality, S is equal to the number
who die by age i ($I\text{-}S_i$) rather than those who survive.

through age five, after which they have a pattern of medical care utilization similar to the general population. Hypothetical data are presented in Table 2-3 on the incremental cost of medical care for those born with this particular birth defect. The data in columns 2-4 of the table relate to the prevalent population with the disease in a particular year. The prevalent population at each age (column 3) depends on the size of the birth cohort, the mortality experience of the cohort, and migration patterns. The fact that there are ten more five than four year-olds with the disease could, therefore, reflect any combination of larger birth cohort size, lower mortality, or greater in-migration into or lower out-migration from the area of study among the five-year-old cohort. Total medical costs reported in column 2 are total incremental medical costs incurred by the prevalent population at each age, whereas column 4 reports average per-capita medical costs, which is the simple division of row entries in column 2 by corresponding entries in column 3.

Cohort data, which are required for the incidence approach that we undertook, are presented in columns 5 and 6 of Table 2-3. The estimate of cohort size at birth (I) in a particular year is presented as the first entry of column 5; succeeding entries in the column (S_i)

Table 2-3. An illustration of the cost of medical care under the incidence approach using hypothetical data on the prevalent and incident populations

Age (years) (1)	Prevalent population data			Cohort data	
	Total medical costs ($) (TCPREV$_i$) (2)	Prevalent population (PREVPOP$_i$) (3)	Per-capita costs ($) (PCPREV$_i$) ((2)x(3)) (4)	Survivors (S_i) (5)	Total cohort medical costs ($) (TC$_i$) ((4)x(5)) (6)
<1	2,400,000	120	20,000	100	2,000,000
1	1,650,000	110	15,000	90	1,350,000
2	720,000	120	6,000	85	510,000
3	380,000	95	4,000	82	328,000
4	237,000	95	2,500	80	200,000
5	105,000	105	1,000	80	80,000

progressively decline, reflecting projected future mortality among this cohort. Per-capita estimates from column 4 ($PCPREV_i$) are multiplied by these estimates of survivors to yield the age-specific total medical cost estimates of interest (TC_{ij}) in column 6 (Equation 2-3). The total cost of medical care for the cohort is the summation of entries in this column after appropriate discounting according to Equation 2-1. At a 4% discount rate, for example, the projected $80,000 in medical costs incurred by the cohort at age five adds $65,754 ($80,000/1.04^5$) to the total incremental medical costs of this birth defect.

We estimated direct medical care costs and indirect mortality costs using Equation 2-3.[f] We could not estimate other direct costs and indirect morbidity costs from Equation 2-3 because $TCPREV_{ij}$ or $PCPREV_{ij}$ could not be obtained directly from available data. Instead, we focused on the "affected" portion of the prevalent population (AFFPOP), which includes all persons with the condition who require incremental services or who suffer from work limitations. Because the impact on health and functioning of any given birth defect varies across individuals and over time, some individuals with a defect require more direct services or have more impaired productivity than others of the same age. Indeed, some individuals with a defect may be "unaffected" at a given age; that is, their service requirements or productivity equal the "average" person in society. Per-capita costs among the "affected" prevalent population (PCAFF), coupled with an estimate of the proportion of the prevalent population "affected," can be used to estimate total costs (TC_{ij}), as expressed in Equation 2-4:

$$TC_{ij} = (S_i) \times (p_{ij}) \times (PCAFF_{ij}), \qquad\qquad [2\text{-}4]$$

where p_{ij} is the proportion of the prevalent population at age i "affected," in the sense described above, with respect to the jth resource, and $PCAFF_{ij}$ is the per-capita incremental cost or value of this jth resource in this population at age i. Because $p_{ij} = AFFPOP_{ij}/PREVPOP_{ij}$ and $PCAFF_{ij}$ is the ratio of total costs among the affected population to that population

---

[f]Estimation of certain long-term care costs for Down syndrome and cerebral palsy, as described in Chapter 4, was made based on Equation 2-5.

$(TCAFF_{ij}/AFFPOP_{ij})$, Equation 2-4 can be rewritten:

$$TC_{ij} = (S_i) \times (AFFPOP_{ij}/PREVPOP_i) \times (TCAFF_{ij}/AFFPOP_{ij}). \quad [2-5]$$

The product of the last two ratios in Equation 2-5 reduces to $(TCAFF_{ij}/PREVPOP_i)$, illustrating the point that Equation 2-5 is simply a restatement of Equation 2-3.[g]

An illustration is provided in Table 2-4 using the same hypothetical cost and population data as in Table 2-3. The entries provided in column 3 of Table 2-4, however, are from the affected rather than the total prevalent population. The proportion affected (p_{ij}) in column 5 is the ratio of the corresponding entries in column 3 of the two tables. All 120 infants less than one year old with the defect incur incremental medical services ($p_{<1} = 1$), for example, whereas only 20% of five year-olds required incremental medical services ($p_5 = .2$). Total cost figures relating to the prevalent population in column 2 of both tables are identical, illustrating the fact that only the affected population generates incremental medical costs. Total medical costs reported for the cohort in the final column of both tables are also the same, demonstrating that Equation 2-5 yields the same results as Equation 2-3. Our estimates of nonmedical direct costs and indirect morbidity costs were based on Equation 2-5. Throughout the remainder of our study, we refer to Equations 2-3 and 2-5 as the "basic equations" or "general formulas" for calculating total cost.

It is readily apparent from the general formulas above that prevalence estimates were required despite our use of the incidence approach. The size of the prevalent population enters the denominator of the last term in Equation 2-3 and the denominator of p (Equation 2-5). Two additional sets of population estimates were required under the incidence approach because the number surviving to each age, S_i, is itself the product of two components:

$$S_i = I \times m_i, \quad [2-6]$$

where I is the number of children born with the birth defect in the base year (the number of "incident" cases) and m_i is an estimate of

---

[g]We note that $TCPREV_{ij} = TCAFF_{ij}$ because, by definition, incremental costs are nonzero only among the subset of the prevalent population that is "affected."

Table 2-4. An illustration of the cost of medical care under the incidence approach using hypothetical data on the "affected" and incident populations

	Prevalent population data				Cohort data	
Age (years) (1)	Total medical costs ($) $(TCAFF_i)$ (2)	Affected population $(AFFPOP_i)$ (3)	Per-capita costs ($) $(PFAFF_i)$ ((2)/(3)) (4)	Proportion affected (a) (p_i) (5)	Survivors (S_i) (6)	Total cohort medical costs (b) ($) (TC_i) ((4)x(5)x(6)) (7)
<1	2,400,000	120	20,000	1.000	100	2,000,000
1	1,650,000	104	15,865	0.945	90	1,350,000
2	720,000	108	6,667	0.900	85	510,000
3	380,000	76	5,000	0.800	82	328,000
4	237,500	62	3,831	0.653	80	200,000
5	105,000	21	5,000	0.200	80	80,000

(a) The proportion affected (p_i) is equal to the affected population in column 3 divided by the prevalent population in column 3 of Table 2-3.

(b) Figures in this column may not equal that provided by the formula because of rounding.

the proportion surviving to age i.[h]

A fundamental challenge in the application of cost-of-illness methodology is merging the general formulas above to what is inevitably imperfect data and doing so in a fashion that entails a minimal amount of compromise of theoretical foundations. A significant portion of the remainder of our study is devoted to a discussion of our specific methodology and the underlying assumptions and limitations in performing this merger of method to data. We provide the specific analytic methods for generating the three sets of general population estimates (incidence (I), survival (m), and prevalence (PREVPOP)) in Chapter 3 and for generating direct and indirect cost estimates (p_{ij} and $PCAFF_{ij}$ or $PCPREV_{ij}$) by cost component, j, in subsequent chapters: Chapter 4 for direct medical

---

[h]In the case of indirect costs due to mortality, I is multiplied by the proportion dying, that is, $1-m_i$.

costs, Chapter 5 for direct nonmedical costs, and Chapter 6 for indirect costs.

Endnotes to Chapter 2

1.Fein R. *Economics of Mental Illness*. New York: Basic Books; 1958.

2.Mushkin SJ, Collings EA. Economic costs of disease and injury. *Public Health Reports*. 1959;74(a):795-809.

3.Rice DP. Estimating the cost of illness. In *Health Economics Series No. 6*. PHS Pub. No. 947-6. Washington, DC: US Government Printing Office; 1966.

4.Weisbrod BA. *Economics of Public Health*. Philadelphia: University of Pennsylvania; 1961.

5.Rice DP, et al. *The Economic Costs of Alcohol and Drug Abuse and Mental Illness: 1985*. Report submitted to the Office of Financing and Coverage Policy of the Alcohol, Drug Abuse, and Mental Health Administration, US Department of Health and Human Services. San Francisco: Institute for Health and Aging, University of California; 1990.

6.Hartunian NS, Smart CN, Thompson MS. *The Incidence and Economic Costs of Major Health Impairments*. Lexington, Massachusetts: DC Heath and Company; 1981.

7.Hu T, Sandifer FH. *Synthesis of Cost of Illness Methodology*. National Center for Health Services Research Contract No. 233-79-3010. Washington, DC: Public Services Laboratory, Georgetown University; 1981.

8.Rice DP, et al. Ibid.

9.Lipscomb J. *Human Capital, Willingness-To-Pay and Cost-Effectiveness Analyses of Screening for Birth Defects in North Carolina*. Durham, North Carolina: Duke University; 1986.

10.Hu T, Sandifer FH. Ibid.

11.Rice DP, Hodgson TA, Kopstein AN. The economic costs of illness: a replication and update. *Health Care Financing Review*. 1985;7(1):61-80.

12.Hartunian NS, et al. Ibid.

13.Rice DP, MacKenzie EJ, and Associates. *Cost of Injury in the United States: A Report to Congress*. San Francisco, California: Institute for Health and Aging, University of California and Injury Prevention Center, The Johns Hopkins University; 1989.

14.Rice DP, et al. Ibid.

15.Hartunian NS, et al. Ibid.

16.Koopman JS, Weed DL. Epigenesis theory: a mathematical model relating causal concepts of pathogenesis in individuals to disease patterns in populations. *American Journal of Epidemiology*. 1990;132:366-390.

17.Ibid.

18.Rice DP, et al. Ibid.

19.National Foundation for Brain Research. *The Cost of Disorders of the Brain*. Washington, DC: Author; 1992.

20.Rice DP, Kelman S. Measuring comorbidity and overlap in the hospitalization cost for alcohol and drug abuse and mental illness. *Inquiry*. 1989;26(2):249-261.

21.National Foundation for Brain Research. Ibid.

22.Ibid.

23.Lipscomb J. Ibid.

24.Hagard S, Carter F, Milne RG. Screening for spina bifida cystica: a cost-benefit analysis. *Br J Prev Soc Med*. 1976;30:40-53.

25.Croen L, Schulman J, Roeper P. *Birth defects in California: January 1, 1983-December 31, 1986*. Emeryville, California: California Birth Defects Monitoring Program; 1990.

26.Hill LM, Kleinberg F. Effects of drugs and chemicals on the fetus and newborn (first of two parts). *Mayo Clin Proc*. 1984;59:707-716.

27.Balducci J, Rodis JF, Rosengren S, Vintzileos AM, Spivey G, Vosseller C. Pregnancy outcome following first-trimester varicella infection. *Obstetr Gynecol*. 1992;79:5-6.

28.Tikkanen J, Heinonen OP. Maternal hyperthermia during pregnancy and cardiovascular malformations in the offspring. *Eur J Epidemiol*. 1991;7:628-635.

29.Milunsky A, Ulcickas M, Rothman KJ, Willett W, Jick SS, Jick H. Maternal heat exposure and neural tube defects. *JAMA*. 1992;268:882-885.

30.Hanson JW, Jones KL, Smith DW. Fetal alcohol syndrome: experience with 41 patients. *JAMA*. 1976;235:1458-1460.

31.Stevenson RE, Burton OM, Ferlauto GJ, Taylor HA. Hazards of oral anticoagulants during pregnancy. *JAMA*. 1980;243:1549-1551.

32.Chavez GF, Mulinare J, Cordero JF. Maternal cocaine use during early pregnancy as a risk factor for congenital urogenital anomalies. *JAMA*. 1989;262:795-798.

33.Drongowski RA, Smith RK Jr, Coran AG, Klein MD. Contribution of demographic and environmental factors to the etiology of gastroschisis: a hypothesis. *Fetal Diag Ther*. 1991;6:14-27.

34.McBride WG. Thalidomide and congenital abnormalities (letter). *Lancet*. 1961;2:1358.

35.Lammer EJ, Cordero JF. Exogenous sex hormone exposure and the risk for major malformations. *JAMA*. 1986;255:3128-3132.

36.Hanson JW, Buehler BA. Fetal hydantoin syndrome: current status. *J Pediatr*. 1982;101:816-818.

37.Spina bifida in infants of women treated with carbamazepine during pregnancy. *N Engl J Med*. 1991;324:674-677.

38.Cordier S, Ha MC, Ayme S, Goujard J. Maternal occupational exposure and congenital malformations. *Scand J Work Environ Health*. 1992;18:11-17.

39.Tikkanen J, Heinonen OP. Risk factors for conal malformations of the heart. *Eur J Epidemiol*. 1992;8:48-57.

40.Schwartz DA, LoGerfo JP. Congenital limb reduction defects in the agricultural setting. *Am J Public Health*. 1988;78:654-658.

41.Miller E, Hare JW, Cloherty JP, et al. Elevated maternal hemoglobin A_{1C} in early pregnancy and major congenital anomalies in infants of diabetic mothers. *N Engl J Med*. 1981;304:1331.

42.Rose BI, Graff S, Spencer R, Hensleigh P, Fainstat T. Major congenital anomalies in infants and glycosylated hemoglobin levels in insulin-requiring diabetic mothers. *J Perinatol*. 1988;8:309-311.

43.MRC Vitamin Study Research Group. Prevention of neural tube defects: Results of the Medical Research Council Vitamin Study. *Lancet*. 1991;338:131-137.

44.Smithells RW, Sheppard S, Schorah CJ, et al. Apparent prevention of neural tube defects by periconceptional multivitamin supplementation. *Arch Dis Child*. 1981;56:911-918.

45.Smithells RW, Seller MJ, Harris R, Fielding DW, Schorah CJ, Nevin NC, et al. Further experience of vitamin supplementation for prevention of neural tube defect recurrences. *Lancet*. 1983;1:1027-1031.

46.Laurence KM, James N, Miller MH, Tennant GB, Campbell H. Double-blind randomized controlled trial of folate treatment before conception to prevent recurrence of neural-tube defects. *Br Med J*. 1981;282:1509-1511.

47.Stoll C, Alembik Y, Dott B, Roth MP. Risk factors in limb reduction defects. *Paediatr Perinat Epidemiol*. 1992;6:323-338.

48.Stoll C, Alembik Y, Roth MP, Dott B, Sauvage P. Risk factors in internal urinary system malformations. *Pediatr Nephrol*. 1990;4:319-323.

49.Baird PA, Sadovnick AD, Yee IM. Maternal age and birth defects: A population study. *Lancet*. 1991;337:527-530.

50.Morris CD, Menashe VD. 25-year mortality after surgical repair of congenital heart defect in childhood: a population-based cohort study. *JAMA*. 1991;266:3447-3452.

51.Norwood WI, Dobell AR, Freed MD, Kirklin JW, Blackstone EH, and the Congenital Heart Surgeons Society. Intermediate results of the arterial switch procedure. *J Thorac Cardiovasc Surg*. 1988;96:854-863.

52.Zhao HX, Miller DC, Reitz BA, Shumway NE. Surgical repair of tetralogy of Fallot: long-term follow-up with particular emphasis on late death and reoperation. *J Thorac Cardiovasc Surg*. 1985;89:204-220.

Chapter 3

Incidence, Prevalence, and Survival of Children With Birth Defects

Introduction

This study was designed to estimate the lifetime economic costs associated with the newly diagnosed cases of several major birth defects in California in 1988. California was selected as the area for the analysis because it offers a unique combination of data from different sources about the incidence of birth defects, the utilization of inpatient and outpatient health care, and the costs of special education. The state houses the CBDMP, for example, one the most extensive active surveillance efforts with respect to birth defects in the world. Our use of newly generated CBDMP data on the incidence of birth defects gave an added precision to our cost estimates that could not have been obtained from other data. The base year for our study was 1988 because that was the latest year for which complete population and cost data were available.

Under the incidence approach described in the previous chapter, per-capita costs among the prevalent population provide the basis for estimating costs among the incident cohort with each birth defect. Three sets of general population estimates are required to calculate total costs according to the two basic Equations (2-3 and 2-5) presented there and used throughout the study. These population estimates are, by birth defect, the number of incident cases in the base year (I), age-specific survival rates (m_i), and age-specific prevalence ($PREVPOP_i$). Incidence and survival estimates are required to estimate the number of survivors by age (S_i) in the two basic equations ($S_i = I \times m_i$), whereas prevalence estimates are required for estimating age-specific per-capita costs ($PCPREV_i$) in those equations. In this chapter, we describe how we used the available data to generate these three sets of population estimates, along with some of the underlying methodological assumptions and potential limitations in this linkage. The resulting population estimates are presented as well.

Incident Cases (I)

In most areas of epidemiology, it is conventional to describe newly diagnosed cases of a condition as *incident* cases. The incidence rate (Ir) is then defined as the number of incident cases (I) over a period of time, divided by the number of persons at risk during that time period (RISKPOP), or

$$Ir = I/(RISKPOP). \qquad [3-1]$$

Alternatively, the number of incident cases is the rate (Ir) multiplied by the population at risk:

$$I = Ir \times (RISKPOP). \qquad [3-2]$$

Numerous investigators have pointed out that birth defect "rates" (Ir) are technically "prevalence proportions" rather than incidence rates because the numerator (i.e., the number of new cases) is completely included in the denominator (i.e., the total number of live births) and because the denominator is independent of time.[1,2] In addition, many incident or newly diagnosed cases are spontaneously or therapeutically aborted. Birth defect "rates," in other words, actually represent the point prevalence of the condition at birth. We use the term "incidence" throughout the study to denote such point prevalence, however, in order to maintain the important distinction between cost estimates for a birth cohort under the incidence approach that we adopted and estimates for all persons with the disease at a particular time under the prevalence approach.ᵃ We computed the number of newly diagnosed or "incident" cases (I) of birth defects in California in 1988 based on estimated "prevalence proportions" at birth, as described below.

Incidence rates (Ir) for all birth defects, except cerebral palsy, were derived from 1983-1988 data collected by the CBDMP. Originally authorized by the California legislature in 1982,[3] the CBDMP is currently the largest active surveillance program for congenital anomalies in the world.[4] The ascertainment area included only seven San Francisco Bay area counties in 1983 but, subsequently, expanded to encompass most of the state. The program employs data collection specialists who routinely visit hospitals and genetic centers in which they review facility logs and identify all children up to one year of age who have been diagnosed with reportable conditions.[5] Cases born in military facilities and infants known to have a birth address outside the CBDMP ascertainment area are excluded. The medical charts for each case are reviewed, and diagnostic information is abstracted and coded according to a modified version of the British Pediatric Association classification system. The British Pediatric Association system is structurally similar to, but more precise than, the ICD-9. Registry data are merged with state vital statistics records to provide additional demographic information.

In order to generate stable incidence rates (Ir), we divided the number of cases in the entire CBDMP database from 1983 through 1988 by the total number of live births in participating counties during each county' s period of involvement (N = 1,030,128). Rates were determined separately for male and female infants. These rates were then multiplied by the total number of live births (RISKPOP) that occurred in California in 1988 (N = 272,979 males and N = 260,449 females) in order to estimate the number of incident cases (I) in that year. These estimates are reported in Table 3-1.

Figures in the table confirm that most of these birth defects have significantly higher incidence among males than among females. The number of total estimated incident cases in 1988 in California ranged, in most instances, between 100 and 300. The greatest number of incident cases was an estimated 944 for cleft lip or palate. Truncus arteriosus, a heart defect, had the fewest estimated cases at fifty-six.

ᵃSee Chapter 2 for a discussion of these two approaches.

Table 3-1. Incidence rates (Ir) of major birth defects in California
(1983-1988) from the California Birth Defects Monitoring Program
and estimated number of incident cases (I) in the 1988 statewide
birth cohort by sex

Condition	Males		Females		Total
	Number/1,000 births (Ir)	Incident cases, 1988 (I)	Number/1,000 births (Ir)	Incident cases, 1988 (I)	Incident cases, 1988 (I)
Spina bifida	0.394	108	0.456	119	226
Truncus arteriosus	0.117	32	0.094	24	56
Transposition/DORV	0.606	166	0.374	97	263
Tetralogy of Fallot	0.388	106	0.310	81	187
Single ventricle	0.144	39	0.111	29	68
Cleft lip or palate	1.906	520	1.626	424	944
TE fistula	0.298	81	0.283	74	155
Atresia, small intestine	0.337	92	0.416	108	200
Colorectal atresia	0.517	141	0.388	101	242
Renal agenesis	0.561	153	0.299	78	231
Urinary obstruction	1.416	386	0.647	168	555
Upper-limb reduction	0.462	126	0.414	108	234
Lower-limb reduction	0.241	66	0.187	49	114
Diaphragmatic hernia	0.413	113	0.326	85	198
Gastroschisis	0.298	81	0.211	55	136
Omphalocele	0.201	55	0.181	47	102
Down syndrome	1.027	281	1.065	277	558

Note: The figures are technically birth prevalence rather than incidence rates. Birth prevalence does not include all incident cases because of miscarriage, therapeutic abortion, or spontaneous regression. Our cost analysis ignored such incident cases, however; thus, birth prevalence became a reasonable measure of incidence.

Because the CBDMP ascertainment area in 1988 excluded three major counties in southern California (Riverside, Ventura, and Los Angeles), we were unable to determine the "actual" number of newly diagnosed cases statewide. The resulting estimates might be slightly biased if nonparticipating counties had significantly different prevalence proportions than participating counties in 1988.

Note that the same infant may have multiple defects; thus, the estimates of incident cases in Table 3-1 cannot be added across conditions. According to CBDMP data, approximately 10% of the infants born with one of the defects of interest had at least two defects. In Chapter 7, we provide estimates of aggregate costs across conditions according to an algorithm that considers the existence of multiple defects.

Even though CBDMP provides the best available estimates of the incidence of congenital anomalies in California, several limitations must be acknowledged. First, only live-born children are included in the case-finding process because the number of birth defects among stillborn infants cannot be determined. In addition, fetal deaths at twenty to twenty-seven weeks of gestation are not consistently reported.[6] If birth defects leading to fetal death were included in CBDMP estimates, the actual indirect costs (i.e., loss of economic productivity) would exceed those estimated in this report. On the other hand, the direct medical costs incurred by stillborn infants are probably modest. Another limitation is that certain internal defects such as renal dysgenesis may not be apparent during the first year of life. If all infants were evaluated radiographically for these conditions, the CBDMP's birth prevalence estimates might be substantially higher. Finally, the CBDMP does not capture birth defects not listed in medical records or diagnosed and treated exclusively on an outpatient basis. Because this cost study is limited to "major" defects that are almost invariably diagnosed or treated in the inpatient setting, resulting bias from this source of error should be insignificant.

Because cerebral palsy is not a structural anomaly manifest at birth, the number of incident cases could not be estimated in the same manner as for the other defects. Instead, we used figures generated by the California Cerebral Palsy Project, which is a CBDMP-administered study of children with moderate to severe congenital cerebral palsy in four San Francisco Bay area counties. In the California Cerebral Palsy Project, cerebral palsy is defined as "a chronic disability of central nervous system origin characterized by aberrant control of movement or posture." This definition specifically excludes acquired cerebral palsy because of infection or head trauma, isolated hypotonia, motor abnormalities due to mental deficiency, and transient or late-appearing disabilities. Cases were identified through review of service records of the California Children' s Services and the California Department of Developmental Services (DDS). Prior fieldwork indicated that these agencies enroll all children in the study counties with moderate or severe congenital cerebral palsy. Case ascertainment for the California Cerebral Palsy Project was limited to children born in 1983 through 1985 who were alive and residing in California at the age of three years. All presumptive cases were linked to vital statistics records to verify that the maternal residence at birth was within the study area. Medical records of these cases were reviewed extensively, and the parents were interviewed. Whenever possible, a California Cerebral Palsy Project physician who was blinded to the medical history confirmed the diagnosis of cerebral palsy through detailed examination and functional assessment of the most affected limb.

The California Cerebral Palsy Project study generated estimates for moderate-to-severe cerebral palsy of 1.36 per 1,000 male survivors and 1.10 per 1,000 female survivors at age three years. These proportions were multiplied by the actual number of live births that occurred in California in 1988. The resulting total represents the number of children from the 1988 birth cohort who would be expected to manifest moderate-to-severe cerebral palsy by the age of three years (the earliest age at which reliable ascertainment is possible).

We used California Cerebral Palsy Project data to estimate the number of cerebral palsy cases diagnosed in the 1988 birth cohort because these data are recent, specific to California, and reflect conservative diagnostic criteria. The California Cerebral Palsy Project estimate is lower than that reported in other population-based studies (summarized in Table 3-2) from Australia, Finland, Great Britain, the United States, and Sweden.[7,8,9,10,11,12,13,14,15] This discrepancy reflects the exceptionally stringent criteria for including cases in the California Cerebral Palsy Project. Few other population-based prevalence studies have excluded all children with acquired or late-appearing cerebral palsy and those without significant functional impairment ("mild" cerebral palsy). The California Cerebral Palsy Project also excluded five children with documented cerebral palsy whose birth residence could not be confirmed and eighteen children with possible cerebral palsy who died or moved out-of-state before their third birthday. If all of these cases had been included, the

Table 3-2. Incidence or prevalence estimates of cerebral palsy from recent population-based studies in developed nations

Study (birth years)	Prevalence proportion (number/1,000)	Comments
California Cerebral Palsy Project (1983-1985) [16]	1.23	Excluded mild or acquired cerebral palsy (based on parent interview and examination)
Western Australia Cerebral Palsy Register (1956-1981) [17,18]	2.50	No consistent change over time
Northern Finland study (1966) [19]	4.20	Excluded cerebral palsy because of degenerative disorders, central nervous system malformations, chromosomal aberrations, or postnatal
Southeast Thames Regional Health Authority (1970-1974) [20]	2.20	Definitions unclear
British Births study (1970) [21]	2.50	Follow-up study of all persons born in the United Kingdom between April 5 and April 11, 1970 (excluded acquired cerebral palsy)
US Collaborative Perinatal Project (1959-1966) [22]	2.60	After excluding mild cases and cases not clearly congenital
Mersey (United Kingdom) study (1967-1984) [23]	1.70	Excluded acquired cerebral palsy
Western Sweden study (1974-1978) [24]	2.00	Retrospective review of hospital records, confirmed by examination

California Cerebral Palsy Project rate would have been 1.38 per 1,000 survivors.

Age-Specific Prevalence (PREVPOP$_i$)

Age-specific prevalence estimates (PREVPOP$_i$) were necessary only up to the age beyond which individuals with a birth defect would be expected to generate negligible incremental costs. For children born with birth defects listed in quadrant I of Table 2-2, excepting those born with colorectal atresia, this threshold was set at twenty-four months of age.[b] Small intestinal atresia and stenosis has an early cutoff because it is uniformly corrected in infancy, whereas colorectal atresia may not be definitively repaired until later in childhood. In children with the latter condition, reanastomosis may be performed months or years after a diverting colostomy; thus, the age cutoff for incremental medical services was set at seventeen years. Urinary obstruction has a twenty-four-month age cutoff because children with this condition receive surgery soon after diagnosis, and our CBDMP-based estimate of the 1988 birth cohort includes only cases diagnosed before one year of age. For those born with all other defects, positive incremental costs were expected to be incurred through adulthood. These age cutoffs were based on literature review and consultation with our panel of clinician advisors; but, in certain instances, as discussed in Chapter 2, they reflected limitations in our data.

Whereas the conditions with early cutoffs listed in quadrant I of Table 2-2 (e.g., gastroschisis, omphalocele, intestinal atresia, tracheoesophageal fistula, and diaphragmatic hernia) are characterized by early surgical intervention and excellent outcomes among children who survive the perioperative period, the conditions with no age cutoff (e.g., cerebral palsy, Down syndrome, spina bifida, cardiac anomalies, and limb reductions) are characterized by lifelong medical care, increased susceptibility to acute medical problems (e.g., urinary tract infections), and an above-average prevalence of disability with respect to school and work. To the extent that children with one of the former conditions actually continue to use more health care or other services than the average child as they grow older, our total estimates of direct costs may be too low. Because many unilateral obstructive defects of the urinary tract are diagnosed late in childhood, our cost estimates for this condition are undoubtedly conservative.

Four age strata were used in our prevalence estimates $(PREVPOP_i)$: i = zero to one year, two to four years, five to seventeen

---

[b]Even though estimates of indirect mortality costs for these defects are based on productivity loss over the entire life span, prevalence estimates are required only to compute the number of excess deaths during the period for which excess mortality is assumed. For defects in quadrant I of Table 2-2, that period is the first year (Chapter 2).

years, and eighteen years or more. These strata reflect critical developmental stages for growing children and transitions between different patterns of service utilization. For example, nearly all surgically correctable defects (except certain cardiac conditions) are operated upon during the first two years of life. The vast majority of all school-based special education services are provided to children five to seventeen years of age, whereas labor force participation generally increases dramatically around the age of eighteen years.

Prevalence for Ages Zero to One

We generated estimates of those zero to one year of age alive in 1988 with each birth defect by adding our estimate of the number of incident cases in 1988 in the last column of Table 3-1 to an estimate of the number of survivors in 1988 from the 1987 birth cohort. The number of survivors in 1988 from the 1987 cohort was determined using incidence and one-year survival data from CBDMP. CBDMP staff determined the proportion of affected children in the CBDMP birth registry from 1983-1986 who were still alive one year later through linkage with death certificates compiled by the California Department of Health Services. These twelve-month survival proportions (column 2 of Table 3-3) were multiplied by estimates of the number of infants born with each defect in 1987 (column 1 of Table 3-3), estimated in the same manner as the number of affected births in 1988. The sum of the number of expected survivors among 1987 births and the estimated number of 1988 births represents the total number of zero to one year-olds alive on July 1, 1988. These estimates are presented in column 4 of Table 3-3 and column 1 of Table 3-4.

This method assumes that the defect-specific probability of survival in 1987-1988 was identical to that in 1983-1986. To the extent that survival improved during the period because of recent medical innovations, the number of prevalent cases may be greater (and per-capita costs may be lower) than our estimates. Our method underestimates the number of children who actually used services during calendar year 1988; that is, a child who died before July 1st might have received substantial care. However, infant deaths occur disproportionately during the first few months of life. We also assumed that first-year mortality was equal among male and female infants. Net migration across state boundaries could not be

Table 3-3. Estimates of the numbers of zero to one-year-old children in California with major birth defects on July 1, 1988

Condition	Estimated births, 1987 (a)	First-year proportional survival (b)	Estimated births, 1988 (I) (a)	Total zero to one year olds alive July 1, 1988 (c)
Spina bifida	214	0.803	226	398
Truncus arteriosus	53	0.381	56	77
Transposition/DORV	248	0.596	263	411
Tetralogy of Fallot	176	0.757	187	321
Single ventricle	64	0.460	68	98
Cleft lip or palate	891	0.860	944	1,710
TE fistula	146	0.752	155	265
Atresia, small intestine	189	0.908	200	372
Colorectal atresia	229	0.749	242	414
Renal agenesis	218	0.370	231	312
Urinary obstruction	524	0.807	555	978
Upper-limb reduction	221	0.855	234	423
Lower-limb reduction	108	0.812	114	202
Diaphragmatic hernia	187	0.437	198	279
Gastroschisis	129	0.851	136	246
Omphalocele	96	0.619	102	162
Down syndrome	527	0.903	558	1,033

(a) The estimated number of births with each condition was determined by multiplying the CBDMP prevalence by the applicable number of live births in California:

1988   N = 272,979 males; N = 260,449 females; N = 533,428 total

1987   N = 258,568 males; N = 245,087 females; N = 503,655 total.

(b) First-year proportional mortality was determined by linking CBDMP registry data for 1983-1986 with death certificates up to one year after birth. Listed below are the ratios between the number of deaths and the number of live births with each condition.

(c) The number of zero to one year olds alive on July 1, 1988, was determined by adding the estimated number of births in 1988 to the estimated number of 1987 births who survived their first year of life.

Table 3-4. Estimates of the numbers of persons in each category alive in California on July 1, 1988 (PREVPOP$_i$)

| Condition | Age group | | | | Total |
	Zero to one (a)	Two to four (b)	Five to seventeen (b)	Eighteen plus (c)	
Spina bifida	398	493	1,593	6,375	8,859
Truncus arteriosus	77	108	314	1,092	1,591
Transposition/DORV	411	503	1,465	5,091	7,469
Tetralogy of Fallot	321	357	1,041	3,618	5,336
Single ventricle	98	131	381	1,323	1,932
Cleft lip or palate	1,710	2,114	6,675	14,457	24,956
TE fistula	265				
Atresia, small intestine	372				
Colorectal atresia	414	459	1,739		
Renal agenesis	312	451	1,710	6,962	9,435
Urinary obstruction	978				
Upper-limb reduction	423	514	1,620	5,338	7,895
Lower-limb reduction	202	251	792	2,610	3,856
Diaphragmatic hernia	279				
Gastroschisis	246				
Omphalocele	162				
Down syndrome	1,033	1,244	3,945	7,873	14,095
Cerebral palsy	1,269	2,489	7,987	17,000	28,745

(a) The number of zero to one-year-old children with each defect was calculated as shown in Table 3-3.

(b) The number of children in these age groups was not estimated for the following conditions: TE fistula; atresia, small intestine; urinary obstruction; diaphragmatic hernia; gastroschisis; and omphalocele. These conditions are characterized by definitive surgical repair in infancy, after which medical care utilization is expected to be normal (in the absence of associated defects). For some of these conditions, there is apparent confusion between congenital and acquired ICD-9-CM codes on hospital discharge abstracts. As a result, adults or older children with these diagnoses (e.g., intestinal stenoses) must be treated as miscodes.

(c) The number of adults was not estimated for the following conditions: TE fistula; atresia, small intestine; colorectal atresia; urinary obstruction; diaphragmatic hernia; gastroschisis; and omphalocele. These conditions are characterized by definitive surgical repair in childhood, after which medical care utilization is expected to be normal (in the absence of associated defects).

estimated. If families with affected children tend to migrate to California because of the availability of specialized services, our prevalence estimates may be too low.

The CBDMP-based infant mortality estimates in Table 3-3 used in this analysis are similar to those previously reported for some conditions but are substantially higher for others. The twelve-month mortality of 9.7% for Down syndrome, for example, is less than the 12.4% reported from the British Columbia registry (1908-1981)[25] and the 13% reported from Queensland (1976-1985)[26] but is greater than the 6.4% reported from Japan (1966-1975).[27] The twelve-month mortality of 56.3% for congenital diaphragmatic hernia is comparable to that reported from several centers in the 1980s.[28,29,30,31] However, survival may have improved significantly since then with the advent of extracorporeal membrane oxygenation.[32,33] Most surprising are the twelve-month mortality proportions of 14% for cleft deformities and 14.5% to 18.7% for limb reductions, neither of which are life-threatening defects. Many of these children are presumably dying from associated anomalies. In attributing their resource utilization to these primary defects, we may have overestimated the potential savings from preventing these defects.[c]

Prevalence After Age One

We were not able to obtain linked data from the CBDMP registry to investigate deaths after twelve months of age. Attempted analysis of unlinked death certificates was unsuccessful because coding congenital anomalies appeared to be unreliable. In addition, we were concerned that in-migration to California might inflate the population of older children and adults with birth defects, which would lead us to overestimate per-capita medical care costs if we derived overall prevalence estimates solely from life-table analyses of earlier birth cohorts. We, therefore, used five years (1985-1989) of pooled data from the National Health Interview Survey, which is an ongoing probability sample of the noninstitutionalized civilian population of the United States to estimate the prevalent population after one year

---

[c]See Chapter 2 for a discussion of the treatment of associated conditions in this and other cost-of-illness studies.

of age. The National Health Interview Survey is a personal household survey, with interviewers requesting information from all family members using proxy respondents for persons less than nineteen years of age. No other data set offers such detailed information about chronic conditions in a large, representative sample with a response rate of more than 95% and extensive procedures for verification and quality assessment. All National Health Interview Survey respondents are asked a set of questions about household composition, demographic characteristics, general health status, limitations of activities, days confined to bed, sick days, hospitalizations, and physician visits. Condition prevalence estimates can be generated from the weighted responses to six specific checklists organized by body system. Each checklist is administered to a one-sixth subsample of the entire National Health Interview Survey sample, consisting of approximately 100,000 persons each year.[34] Sample weights correct for the complex multistage sampling design and the oversampling of Black households in the National Health Interview Survey. Because congenital anomalies are relatively rare, we pooled five years of National Health Interview Survey data to generate more stable estimates of age-specific prevalence. The a and b parameters provided by the National Center for Health Statistics were used to estimate the variance of each prevalence estimate.

The National Center for Health Statistics aggregates all chronic conditions and impairments to 134 categories, known as "Diagnostic Recode C," which are designed to be sufficiently broad to provide reliable prevalence estimates.[d] Among these categories are several major birth defects, including spina bifida, cerebral palsy, cleft lip or palate, missing extremities, absent kidney, and congenital heart disease.[e] A single National Health Interview Survey cannot be used

---

[d]According to the National Center for Health Statistics, "The data collection and coding procedures used do not justify any further breakdown of categories for purposes of estimating prevalence."

[e]Several ICD-9-coded diseases are grouped on the National Health Interview Survey into special "X" categories, and several of the Recode "C" categories are comprised of one or several of these X codes. X codes are designated with a trailing digit of "9" on the National Health Interview Survey when they are reported to be

to estimate reliably the prevalence of conditions that are subsets of a broader "Recode C" code category such as urinary tract obstruction.

Accordingly, we estimated the population prevalence of each congenital anomaly for which a corresponding Recode C was available in the National Health Interview Survey, by age stratum (zero to one, two to four, five to seventeen, and greater than seventeen years). These prevalence estimates were based on a relatively large number of respondents with cerebral palsy (N=277), intermediate numbers with spina bifida (N=118) and cleft lip or palate (N=94), and small numbers with missing extremities (N=59) and absent kidneys (N=38). For each of these conditions, the majority of affected respondents were adults, and relatively few were in the two youngest age strata. We, therefore, had more confidence in the prevalence estimates for adults than in those for children.

The adult prevalence proportions computed from the National Health Interview Survey were multiplied by the number of adult residents in California on July 1, 1988, according to intercensal population estimates from the US Bureau of the Census.[35] In so doing, we assumed that each condition' s prevalence in California is similar to its prevalence nationwide. This assumption may be invalid if California selectively attracts families with affected children from other states because of superior educational and medical services. However, no evidence is available to support this hypothesis.

The number of adults with spina bifida, cerebral palsy, congenital missing kidneys (renal agenesis), and cleft deformities was derived directly from the National Health Interview Survey Recode C prevalence estimates. This simple estimation procedure was impossible for upper and lower limb reductions and specific congenital heart defects because the Recode C categories were too broad; for example, all congenital heart disease was assigned to one Recode C category, as were all congenital and noncongenital limb reductions. For these two conditions, we allocated affected adults to individual subgroups based on the proportionate distribution of these defects at birth reported by the CBDMP. For example, 452 of the 638 (70.8%) infants with limb reductions in the CBDMP data set (1983-1988) had upper-limb deformities, whereas 221 (34.6%) had

---

congenital.

lower-limb deformities.[36] The frequency estimates in Table 3-4 were generated by applying these percentages to the estimated total of 7,535 adults in California with limb reductions. Similarly, 1.9% of all infants with congenital heart disease in the CBDMP data set had truncus arteriosus, 8.8% had transposition of the great vessels, 6.3% had tetralogy of Fallot, and 2.3% had single ventricle. The frequency estimates in Table 3-4 were generated by applying these percentages to the estimated total of 57,811 adults in California with congenital heart disease from the National Health Interview Survey. This estimation procedure assumes that the distribution of limb deformities and congenital heart disease across subtypes remains constant with age. This assumption is questionable because specific subtypes have higher mortality than others, and minor conditions are, therefore, likely to be overrepresented among older individuals.

The frequencies of major defects in the younger age groups (two to four and five to seventeen years) could not be reliably estimated directly from the National Health Interview Survey Recode C prevalence estimates because of small numbers of respondents in those age groups. The prevalence estimates by age stratum showed excessive variability. We, therefore, imputed prevalence values from a quadratic smoothing function estimated using weighted least squares. The dependent variable in each model was the age-specific, weighted prevalence proportion from the National Health Interview Survey (cases per 1,000 population), and the independent variables were age (the midpoint of each age group) and age squared. Each observation in these models represented an age stratum: two to nine, ten to seventeen, eighteen to twenty-four, twenty-five to thirty-four, thirty-five to forty-four, forty-five to fifty-four, and more than fifty-five years. These strata were defined to have approximately equal numbers of the National Health Interview Survey respondents. Observations were weighted by the inverse of the estimated variance, which was calculated using parameters provided by the National Center for Health Statistics. Each equation was forced through a point representing the number of affected zero to one year-olds in California estimated from the CBDMP birth prevalence and first-year survival data.[f] Because CBDMP data are specific to California and

---

[f]Further details regarding the smoothing functions can be obtained on request from the authors.

are based on active surveillance rather than self-report, we were more confident in our prevalence estimates for zero to one year-olds than in those for older children and adults. As expected, the estimated prevalences of all conditions decrease with age because of premature mortality (or response bias, if older respondents fail to recall their congenital anomalies).

Just as for adults, we multiplied the prevalence proportions computed from the National Health Interview Survey (after imputation using the smoothing functions described above) by the number of California residents in each analytic age group (two to four and five to seventeen years) on July 1, 1988, according to intercensal population estimates from the US Bureau of the Census.[37] In so doing, we assumed that each condition's prevalence in California is similar to its prevalence nationwide. For limb reductions and congenital heart disease, we again allocated the total number of estimated cases to clinical subgroups (e.g., upper versus lower limb, truncus arteriosus versus transposition) based on the birth prevalence proportions reported by the CBDMP.

Two conditions (Down syndrome and colorectal atresia) were aggregated into such broad "C" categories (mental retardation and gastrointestinal anomalies, respectively) that the National Health Interview Survey data could not be used reliably to estimate their prevalences. Instead, we used a life-table approach based on estimating survival from previous birth cohorts for estimating prevalence after age one year. The number of births with Down syndrome in each year, going back to 1905, was estimated by multiplying the total number of California births recorded in that year by the incidence of Down syndrome among 1983-1988 live births from the CBDMP. The survival rates reported by Baird and Sadovnick from the British Columbia registry[38] then were applied to estimate the number of persons from each birth cohort who would still be living in 1988. Baird and Sadovnick's life table was modified slightly by decreasing first-year mortality from 12.4% to 9.7% in accordance and with California data provided by the CBDMP. For example, we estimated that 292 of the 389 persons with Down syndrome believed to have been born in 1960 would still have been alive in 1988 (at the age of twenty-eight years). The total number of living persons with Down syndrome in each analytic age group was estimated by adding the numbers of expected survivors from all relevant birth cohorts. A similar approach was employed for colorectal atresia, except that mortality was assumed to be the same as that of the general population after twelve months of age. Gender-specific life tables for the general population in 1988 were applied to the expected number of first-year survivors with colorectal atresia from each birth cohort back to 1905.[39]

This approach assumes no net migration and no change in mortality over time. Even though neither of these assumptions is valid, the resulting errors may cancel out because migration presumably has increased the number of affected adults and older children in California, whereas higher mortality in earlier decades presumably has decreased the number of affected adults. The life-table approach to estimating current prevalences also assumes that the prevalence of each defect at birth has been constant over time. According to the CBDMP, the birth prevalence of Down syndrome and colorectal atresia did not change between 1984 and 1988. This stability is reassuring but cannot necessarily be extrapolated backward to a time when women bore children at earlier ages and genetic screening of fetuses by amniocentesis was impossible. Selective termination of fetuses with Down syndrome theoretically could affect the prevalence of the condition at birth.[g]

Age-Specific Survival Proportion (m$_i$)

Finally, we estimated age-specific survival proportions (m$_i$) for children with major birth defects. These estimates, coupled with estimates of incident cases (I) in the 1988 birth cohort, provide the foundation for computing the numbers of survivors (S$_i$) and decedents (I-S$_i$) at each age, i, used to estimate costs attributable to birth defects according to the basic equations presented in Chapter 2. A life table was created for each condition based on information from

---

[g]As explained above, we were hesitant to rely on aggregate National Health Interview Survey recodes to make prevalence estimates for Down syndrome. However, an estimate of the percentage of the congenitally mentally retarded with Down syndrome at birth was available. Multiplying this percentage by the X and Recode C categories (congenital mental retardation) on the National Health Interview Survey into which it was folded in the adult population yielded prevalence estimates that were surprisingly close to (within 3% of) the estimate from the life table.

three sources. Resultant estimates of the number of survivors at selected ages (S_i) are provided in Table 3-5.

As described above with respect to estimates of prevalence among zero to one year-olds, first-year mortality was derived from the CBDMP's linkage of 1983-1986 registry records with death certificates. The CBDMP data were used to estimate first-year mortality because they reflect community experience throughout California. The precipitous decline in survival between age 0 and 1 year in Table 3-5 for many of the defects reflects data from the CBDMP registry. The subsequent leveling off of survival for those born with defects listed in quadrants I and II of Table 2-2 reflects our assumption that mortality nearly reverts back to normal for individuals with such defects.

For conditions in quadrant IV of Table 2-2 in which mortality would be expected to remain significantly higher than normal beyond the first year of life, we estimated subsequent survival from detailed review of the clinical literature. A MEDLINE search was conducted for each condition using survival and mortality as key words, focusing on articles published in English language journals since 1980. In general, we obtained survival estimates from the largest identified study with a representative sample and suitable long-term follow-up. We attempted to avoid relying on studies from referral centers in favor of studies from population registries. When no studies were available such as congenital heart defects, we used meta-analytic techniques to combine a multiple series of comparable value from different centers weighting each series by its sample size. Because mortality rates were rarely reported separately by gender, we generally assumed that males and females had equal defect-related mortality.

Finally, gender-specific life tables for the general population were used to estimate survival for each condition beyond the age at which excess mortality would be expected to disappear. The underlying assumption is that, for each birth defect, there is a discrete point beyond which survivors have mortality rates resembling that of the general population. These points were determined by review of the clinical literature and discussion with our panel of clinical advisors. For several conditions such as spina bifida and renal agenesis, there is reason to suspect excess mortality throughout life; but no studies in the clinical literature provide sufficiently long follow-up to quantify survival into adulthood. In the absence of data, we assumed that mortality rates were equivalent to those of the gender and age-matched population of the United States.

Our three-part approach to estimating survival among affected persons born in 1988 suffers from several sources of bias. First, actual first-year mortality among affected children born in 1988 may have been less than comparable mortality in 1983-1986 when the CBDMP linkage with death certificates was performed. Similarly, postinfant mortality among affected children born in 1988 may be less than that reported in clinical series from the early-to-mid 1980s. These biases would lead us to underestimate the number of survivors and, hence, exaggerate the indirect costs resulting from premature death. However, an opposing bias results from the assumption of normal mortality beyond a specific age. If excess mortality persists beyond that age, then we may have overestimated the number of survivors and, hence, understated the indirect costs resulting from premature death.

Table 3-5. Estimated number of survivors (S^i) at selected ages from the 1988 California cohort of live births with each congenital anomaly by sex

Condition	Male survivors at age						
	0	1	2	5	17	45	65
Spina bifida	108	86	85	82	81	76	61
Truncus arteriosus	32	12	12	12	12	11	9
Transposition/DORV	166	99	99	98	98	92	73
Tetralogy of Fallot	106	80	80	80	80	75	60
Single ventricle	39	18	18	18	18	17	13
Cleft lip or palate	520	447	447	446	444	417	333
TE fistula	81	61	61	61	61	57	45
Atresia, small intestine	92	84	84	83	83	78	62
Colorectal atresia	141	106	106	106	105	99	79
Renal agenesis	153	57	57	57	56	53	42
Urinary obstruction	386	312	312	311	310	291	232
Upper-limb reduction	126	108	108	108	107	101	80
Lower-limb reduction	66	53	53	53	53	50	40
Diaphragmatic hernia	113	49	49	49	49	46	37
Gastroschisis	81	69	69	69	69	64	51
Omphalocele	55	34	34	34	34	32	25
Down syndrome	280	253	242	234	220	197	76
Cerebral palsy	371	367	363	351	328	308	245

Table 3-5. (Continued)

	Female survivors at age						
	0	1	2	5	17	45	65
Spina bifida	119	95	94	91	90	87	77
Truncus arteriosus	24	9	9	9	9	9	8
Transposition/DORV	97	58	58	58	58	56	50
Tetralogy of Fallot	81	61	61	61	61	59	52
Single ventricle	29	13	13	13	13	13	11
Cleft lip or palate	424	364	364	363	362	353	311
TE fistula	74	55	55	55	55	54	47
Atresia, small intestine	108	98	98	98	98	95	84
Colorectal atresia	101	76	76	76	75	73	65
Renal agenesis	78	29	29	29	29	28	25
Urinary obstruction	168	136	136	136	135	132	116
Upper-limp reduction	108	92	92	92	92	89	79
Lower-limb reduction	49	40	40	40	39	38	34
Diaphragmatic hernia	85	37	37	37	37	36	32
Gastroschisis	55	47	47	47	47	45	40
Omphalocele	47	29	29	29	29	28	25
Down syndrome	277	251	240	231	218	195	75
Cerebral palsy	286	283	280	271	253	246	217

Table 3-5. (Continued)

	Total survivors at age						
	0	1	2	5	17	45	65
Spina bifida	226	182	178	173	170	163	137
Truncus arteriosus	56	21	21	21	21	20	17
Transposition/DORV	263	157	156	156	156	148	123
Tetralogy of Fallot	187	141	141	141	141	134	112
Single ventricle	68	31	31	31	31	30	25
Cleft lip or palate	944	811	811	810	807	770	644
TE fistula	155	116	116	116	116	111	93
Atresia, small intestine	200	182	182	182	181	173	146
Colorectal atresia	242	181	181	181	180	172	143
Renal agenesis	231	85	85	85	85	81	67
Urinary obstruction	555	448	447	447	445	422	348
Upper-limb reduction	234	200	200	200	199	190	159
Lower-limb reduction	114	93	93	93	92	88	74
Diaphragmatic hernia	198	86	86	86	86	82	68
Gastroschisis	136	116	116	116	115	110	91
Omphalocele	102	63	63	63	63	60	50
Down syndrome	558	504	482	465	438	393	151
Cerebral palsy	657	650	643	622	581	553	462

Note: Row totals by age may not equal corresponding row sums because of rounding.

Endnotes to Chapter 3

1.Hook EB. Incidence and prevalence as measures of the frequency of birth defects. *Am J. Epidemiol.* 1982;116:743-747.

2.Schulman J, Shaw G, Selvin S. On "rates" of birth defects. *Teratology.* 1988;38:427-429.

3.204 California Health and Safety Code § 10800-10806.

4.Kizer KW, Ferguson SC, Harris JA. *California's birth defects monitoring program.* Calif Physician. 1989;XX(4):38-41.

5.Croen L, Schulman J, Roeper P. *Birth Defects in California: January 1, 1983-December 31, 1986.* Emeryville, California: California Birth Defects Monitoring Program; 1990.

6.Kelsey JL, Thompson WD, Evans AS. *Methods in Observational Epidemiology.* New York: Oxford University Press; 1986:55.

7.Grether JK, Cummins SK, Nelson KB. The California Cerebral Palsy Project. *Pediatr Perinat Epidemiol.* 1992;in press.

8.Stanley FJ. An epidemiological study of cerebral palsy in Western Australia, 1956-1975. I: Changes in total incidence of cerebral palsy and associated factors. *Develop Med Child Neurol.* 1979;21:701-713.

9.Stanley FJ, Watson L. The cerebral palsies in Western Australia: Trends, 1968 to 1981. *Am J. Obstet Gynecol.* 1988;158:89-93.

10.Von Wendt L, Rantakallio P, Saukkonen AL, Tuisku M, Makinen H. Cerebral palsy and additional handicaps in a 1-year birth cohort from nothern Finland: A prospective follow-up study to the age of 14 years. *Ann Clin Res.* 1985;17:156-161.

11.Evans P, Elliott M, Alberman E, Evans S. Prevalence and disabilities in 4 to 8 year olds with cerebral palsy. *Arch Dis Child.* 1985; 60:940-945.

12.Emond A, Golding J, Peckham C. Cerebral palsy in two national cohort studies. *Arch Dis Child.* 1989;64:848-852.

13.Nelson KB, Ellenberg JH. Epidemiology of cerebral palsy. *Adv Neurol.* 1978;19:421-435.

14.Pharoah POD, Cooke T, Cooke RWI, Rosenbloom L. Birthweight specific trends in cerebral palsy. *Arch Dis Child.* 1990;65:602-606.

15.Hagberg B, Hagberg G, Olow I. The changing panorama of cerebral palsy in Sweden. IV. Epidemiologic trends 1959-78. *Acta Pediatr Scand.* 1984;73:443-440.

16.Grether JK, et al. Ibid.

17.Stanley FJ. Ibid.

18.Stanley FJ, Watson L. Ibid.

19.Von Wendt L, et al. Ibid.

20.Evans P, et al. Ibid.

21.Emond A, et al. Ibid.

22.Nelson KB, Ellenberg JH. Ibid.

23.Pharoah POD, et al. Ibid.

24.Hagberg B, et al. Ibid.

25.Baird PA, Sadovnick AD. Life tables for Down syndrome. *Hum Genet.* 1989;82:291-292.

26.Bell JA, Pearn JH, Firman D. Childhood deaths in Down syndrome. Survival curves and causes of death from a total population study in Queensland, Australia, 1976 to 1985. *J Med Genet.* 1989;26:764-768.

27.Bohn DH, James I, Filler RM, et al. The relationship between $PaCO_2$ and ventilatory parameters: predicting survival in congenital diaphragmatic hernia. *J Pediatr Surg.* 1984;19:666-671.

28.Hansen J, James S, Burrington J, Whitfield J. The decreasing incidence of pneumothorax and improving survival of infants with congenital diaphragmatic hernia. *J Pediatr Surg.* 1984;19:385-388.

29.Masaki M, Higurashi M, Iijima K, Ishikawa N, Tanaka F, Fugii T, et al. Mortality and survival for Down syndrome in Japan. *Am J Hum Genet.* 1981; 33:629-639.

30.Reynolds M, Luck SR, Lappen R. The "critical" neonate with diaphragmatic hernia: a 21-year perspective. *J Pediatr Surg.* 1984;19:364-369.

31.Weiner, ES. Congenital diaphragmatic hernia: new dimensions in management. *Surgery.* 1982;92:670-681.

32.Heiss K, Manning P, Oldham KT, Coran AG, Polley TZ, Wesley JR, et al. Reversal of mortality for congenital diaphragmatic hernia with ECMO. *Ann Surg.* 1989;209:225-230.

33.Weber TR, Connors RH, Pennington DG, Westfall S, Keenan W, Kotagal S, et al. Neonatal diaphragmatic hernia: an improving outlook with extracorporeal membrane oxygenation. *Arch Surg.* 1987;122:615-618.

34.Adams PF, Benson V. *Current Estimates From the National Health Interview Survey, 1989.* Vital Health Stat, Series 10, No. 176. Hyattsville, Maryland: National Center for Health Statistics; 1990.

35.US Bureau of the Census. *Current Population Reports.* Series P-25, No. 1044.

36.Ibid.

37.Ibid.

38.Baird PA, Sadovnick AD. Ibid.

39.National Center for Health Statistics. *Vital Statistics of the United States, 1988, Vol. II, Mortality, Part A.* DHHS Publication No. (PHS) 91-1101. Washington, DC: Public Health Service; 1991.

Chapter 4

The Direct Medical Costs of Birth Defects

Introduction

The diverse array of medical care that is often required for infants born with each defect was described in some detail in Chapter 2 and in greater detail in Appendix 1. Successful corrective surgery in infancy is critical to survival or to the restoration and maintenance of function in the case of several birth defects. Such surgery can be very expensive. In the case of individuals with heart defects, for example, it is not uncommon for surgical care to cost several hundred thousand dollars by the end of the first year of life. Associated infections with several conditions also may require inpatient stays beyond that of the "average" child. Special appliances and prostheses are often required for those with spina bifida, limb reductions, and cerebral palsy, as is long-term care for those with the severest cases of Down syndrome, cerebral palsy, and other congenital anomalies.

This chapter is devoted to our estimates of direct medical costs of birth defects. We describe our application of the general methodology provided in Chapter 2 to the calculation of these costs and present our final estimates. Relevant categories of service include inpatient care, outpatient care, pharmaceuticals, laboratory tests, x-rays, appliances, and long-term care.

General Method

The method for estimating direct medical costs of birth defects under the incidence approach adopted for this study involves making an estimate of the incremental medical costs over the life span for the cohort that newly contracts the condition of interest in the base year: 1988. Because our study examines costs associated with birth defects, we estimated this medical cost profile for a birth cohort (those born in 1988) with each condition. Estimated medical costs incurred after the first year of life are discounted back to birth, reflecting the tenet in economics that current resources are more highly valued than resources in the future.[a]

Some useful typologies of birth defects for calculating their costs were provided in Table 2-2. As described in more detail in Chapter 2, we estimated medical costs through the second year of life only for all conditions listed in quadrant I of Table 2-2 except colorectal atresia. Estimation of costs through the second year reflected the fact that early surgical correction and medical care for infants with these defects generally restore normal function; thus, the incremental costs of medical care after the second year is minimal. Medical costs for those with colorectal atresia were estimated through age seventeen, however, reflecting our expectation of greater than average medical care utilization through that age for this condition. For all other conditions, we estimated medical costs through age sixty-five. The impact of discounting on total medical costs are, therefore, considerably less for conditions listed in quadrant I of Table 2-2 than for the other conditions.

We used cross-sectional data on medical costs in the prevalent population to estimate the profile of medical costs through the above ages according to Equation 2-3.[b] For each age category and condition, we generated total-cost estimates in the prevalent population (TCPREV) separately for inpatient, outpatient, and long-term care. As described below, we then divided them by estimates of the size of that population (PREVPOP) in 1988 to compute gross

---

[a]See Chapter 2 for a fuller discussion of discounting in cost-of-illness studies.

[b]The calculation of long-term care costs for those with Down syndrome and cerebral palsy was made according to Equation 2-5, as discussed below.

per-capita medical costs in the prevalent population. In order to compute per-capita incremental costs (PCPREV), we subtracted average per-capita medical costs from these gross costs. An assumption in subtracting all medical costs for an average person is that our data captured all medical costs for people with the underlying conditions of interest. It is unlikely that all such costs are truly identifiable from cross-sectional administrative data, but several adjustments were made, as discussed below, to compensate for deficiencies in the available data.

The use of cross-sectional data to approximate the profile of medical costs over a lifetime rests on an underlying assumption that current treatment patterns are representative of future treatment patterns. Medical advances in treatment and/or detection could reduce or increase the actual costs associated with medical care for children born with birth defects in 1988. For example, fetal surgery may decrease the cost of future care for children with congenital diaphragmatic hernia, whereas advances in extracorporeal membrane exaggeration might increase the cost by allowing more children to survive with chronic lung disease that requires continued care. Our estimates should not be affected dramatically by technological changes more than four years hence, however, given that a disproportionate share of medical treatment for several of the birth defects we analyzed is administered in the first few years of life, that is, years that are proximate to the survey year from which we generate cost estimates.

Data

The major sources of data for medical costs were the 1988 California Office of Statewide Health Planning and Development (OSHPD) hospital discharge file and the 1988 MediCal (California' s Medicaid program) "tape-to-tape" file. The OSHPD file contains medical, financial, and demographic data for all discharges from nonfederal hospitals in California and served as the primary data file for calculating inpatient costs of birth defects. The MediCal file similarly contains such information, as well as data on outpatient and long-term care utilization for the MediCal eligible population in California. The file provided the basis for calculating other medical costs. The differences in underlying construction of the two data files, however, presented opportunities for adjusting each medical cost component to better approximate total costs, as discussed below.

Sample Selection

Office of Statewide Health Planning and Development—The OSHPD sample was selected on the basis of a diagnosis of interest, appearing as the principal diagnosis or as a secondary diagnosis in any of the twenty-four available secondary diagnosis fields. Only records from acute-care hospitals were selected. Based on our determination that infants with omphalocele were often incorrectly coded as having umbilical hernias, we selected infants less than one year of age, with the latter diagnosis only if they underwent a surgical procedure for correction of an abdominal wall defect, died, or were transferred to another acute care hospital for definitive management.

Careful analysis of the listed diagnoses and procedures demonstrated that ICD-9 codes for congenital anomalies are incorrectly applied to many hospitalized adults and older children who almost certainly have acquired conditions. For example, we noted a substantial number of adult hospitalizations with the ICD-9 diagnosis code for congenital diaphragmatic hernia. Most of these patients probably had hiatal hernias, a frequent and clinically insignificant condition. Such cases were excluded based on the age cutoffs beyond which children would be expected to utilize no more health care services than the general population. To the extent that incremental medical care actually continued beyond such age cutoffs, we underestimated the medical costs of such conditions in our effort to eliminate costs related to miscoding. Our selection criteria generated more than 20,000 inpatient episodes for our analysis.

In addition to its comprehensiveness in covering all admissions to nonfederal hospitals in California, an obvious strength of the OSHPD file stems from the large number of available diagnosis fields. On the other hand, if a birth defect of interest is considered to be "incidental" to a patient's hospital care or if the recording of diagnoses is simply incomplete, then the selected OSHPD data may contain only a subset of all hospital admissions for people with birth defects of interest.

MediCal—Selection of the MediCal sample was based on a diagnosis of interest (ICD-9 code) appearing in any inpatient, outpatient, or long-term care record in 1988. This selection criterion generated an analytic file of more than 8,000 inpatient records and more than 500,000 outpatient records for a sample of 14,573 individuals with one or more conditions of interest in 1988. The MediCal file lacked the comprehensiveness of the OSHPD sample; that is, only MediCal-covered services for the eligible population were included. In addition, only a single, principal diagnosis for any given service is recorded.

However, the MediCal file had the strength of having a longitudinal component. Once a diagnosis of interest appeared for an individual for any service such as outpatient, inpatient, or long-term care during the year, all MediCal-reimbursed services received by that person during that year were incorporated into the analytic file. Thus, some of the inpatient episodes inappropriately left off of the OSHPD file (because the birth defect diagnosis was not coded on the discharge abstract from that hospitalization) appeared on the MediCal file. On the other hand, if a MediCal-eligible person with a condition of interest received medical services during the year, but the condition was always listed as a secondary and never as the primary diagnosis, then none of those medical services was included in the MediCal sample. Some such hospital episodes may have appeared on the OSHPD file because the birth defect may have been listed as a secondary diagnosis on the corresponding discharge abstract.

Data Reconciliation

Differences in the underlying construction of the OSHPD and McdiCal filcs provided the opportunity for adjustment and reconciliation. Incidental omissions from both files were expected to increase with age as birth defects become less important contributors to the utilization of health care by affected individuals. Furthermore, omissions should be more likely for surgically correctable defects such as cleft lip or palate and intestinal atresia than for chronic uncorrectable defects such as Down syndrome. For these chronic defects and among older patients, hospital episodes appear more likely to be missing in the OSHPD file than in the MediCal file because of the longitudinal linkage of inpatient, outpatient, and long-term care in the latter data set. For example, an adult with congenital heart disease might have one or more outpatient visits related primarily to that condition, but any inpatient episodes may appear to be unrelated. The congenital heart disease would then never appear on OSHPD's discharge abstracts. We, therefore, adjusted the inpatient cost estimates derived from OSHPD data upward for certain defects based upon a comparative analysis with MediCal data, as discussed below.

Estimation of Costs

Inpatient Costs

Given its comprehensiveness in covering all inpatient admissions to nonfederal hospitals in California, the OSHPD file was selected as the primary source of calculating the total inpatient costs of each birth defect (TCPREV). A detailed comparison was made between inpatient admissions, length of stay, and charges where MediCal was listed as the expected principal source of payment on the OSHPD file[c] and the corresponding information on the MediCal file. If both data sets were complete and the expected source of payment was accurately identified on OSHPD records, then the two files would have been identical. In fact, discrepancies were found between the MediCal and OSHPD files for several birth defect categories.

Adjustments were made to the inpatient cost estimates from the OSHPD file based upon this comparative analysis. Condition- and age-specific ratios (CASRs-INP) of total inpatient charges on the MediCal file to total hospital charges on the OSHPD file where MediCal (or "no pay") was listed as the expected payer were computed. These CASRs-INP are provided in Table 4-1. With a few exceptions, the MediCal file included more admissions and higher total charges among affected individuals over one year of age than the corresponding OSHPD file. This discrepancy generally increased

---

[c]We also included charges for those listed as "no pay" on the OSHPD discharge abstract in addition to MediCal in the event that MediCal is the ultimate payer in several such instances. This adjustment created a downward bias in the ratio discussed below based upon the comparison of the two data sets. Resultant cost estimates, therefore, may be downwardly biased.

Table 4-1. Ratios of inpatient charges on the MediCal tape-to-tape file to the California Office of Statewide Health Planning and Development file (a, b, c) (CASRS-INP)

Condition	Age group			
	Zero to one	Two to four	Five to seventeen	Eighteen plus
Spina bifida	1.03	2.54	1.84	2.07
Truncus arteriosus	1.79	12.32	13.85	11.26
Transposition/DORV	.66	1.81	.89	10.71
Tetralogy of Fallot	1.11	1.20	1.81	2.35
Single ventricle	.77	1.47	1.81	17.61
Cleft lip or palate	.99	2.32	2.57	14.41
TE fistula	.77	. .	. .	. .
Atresia, small intestine	.59	. .	. .	. .
Colorectal atresia	.71	5.19	1.75	. .
Renal agenesis	.20	1.32	.20	.97
Urinary obstruction	.24	. .	. .	. .
Upper-limp reduction	.10	.62	1.00	4.71
Lower-limp reduction	.23	1.96	1.04	9.35
Diaphragmatic hernia	.52	. .	. .	. .
Gastroschisis	.83	. .	. .	. .
Down syndrome	.66	1.39	.67	1.80
Cerebral palsy	1.86	1.40	1.21	.98

Note: See Table 1-3 and Appendix 2 for descriptions of these data files.

(a) Charges from the California Office of Statewide Health Planning and Development (OSHPD) file are restricted to those with MediCal or "no pay" as expected source of payment (see text).

(b) Costs of omphalocele were computed only from the OSHPD file. Costs of TE fistula; atresia, small intestine; urinary obstruction; diaphragmatic hernia; and gastroschisis were computed through age one only, whereas colorectal atresia was computed through age seventeen (see text).

(c) These ratios were only used to adjust total costs derived from the OSHPD file when they exceeded one; otherwise, the OSHPD file was assumed to capture all hospitalizations for the condition of interests (see text).

with age, confirming our prior expectations. These ratios formed the basis for constructing condition- and age-specific multipliers to the OSHPD file as follows: (a) if CASR-INP $\leq$ 1, then multiplier = 1 or (b) if CASR-INP > 1, then multiplier = CASR-INP.

The multiplier was applied to all OSHPD charges regardless of the expected source of payment.[d] An underlying assumption of this procedure is that missing MediCal cases on the OSHPD file are comparable to missing cases for which there was a different expected source of payment. We tested this assumption by comparing mean length of stay and mean charges on the OSHPD file, stratified by age group and birth defect category across expected sources of payment. The results of this analysis suggested that inpatient stays paid by MediCal are similar to those paid through private insurance.

Adjustments of charges to cost—Even though many cost-of-illness studies employ charges as a best proxy for costs, charges are not the same as costs. Most payers reimburse hospitals less than their total charges. Under the Medicare program, the Health Care Financing Administration calculates urban and rural hospital ratios of cost-to-charges (RCC) for each state based upon an analysis of local wages and the cost of other resources used in patient care. We adjusted OSHPD charges from OSHPD discharge abstracts downward to estimated cost based upon the weighted average of Medicare' s RCC for California' s rural and urban hospitals, which was .5736 in fiscal year 1988-1989.

This downward adjustment may be too drastic. According to American Hospital Association data that include certain categories of expenses not recognized by Medicare such as nonpatient care activities, Medicare payments were found to be 89% of hospital costs in California in 1989.[1]

---

[d]For admissions paid by health maintenance organizations such as Kaiser, no charge data were listed in the OSHPD data set, although length of stay was reported. We estimated the charges for zero-charge admissions by calculating the product of the mean condition-specific and age-specific per diem charges of all other cases and the total length of stay for zero-charge admissions.

Outpatient Costs

Outpatient costs were estimated based upon condition-specific ratios for each age group of outpatient to inpatient costs (CASRs-OUT) from the MediCal file. These ratios were applied to the total estimated inpatient costs by condition and age to arrive at an estimate of total outpatient costs by condition and age (TCPREV). This method rested on the assumption that the ratio of outpatient to inpatient services for the MediCal-eligible population with birth defects was similar to that of the noneligible population. This assumption seemed reasonable, given the similarity between MediCal and other payers in mean lengths of stay and charges for most birth defects according to the OSHPD database.

In order to calculate reliable CASRs-OUT from the MediCal file, both the numerator (outpatient services) and denominator (inpatient services) had to be expressed in terms, preferably cost, that could be generalized from MediCal to non-MediCal services. Inpatient charges from the MediCal file were adjusted downward to costs using the California Medicare ratios of cost-to-charges, as above. Adjusting the numerator was more difficult because the economic cost of physician services is unknown. Analyses of physician participation in the MediCal program suggest that MediCal generally reimburses physicians under costs and considerably below Medicare-allowable charges, which were 62% of an index of physician fees in 1989.[2] We established Medicare-allowable charges (1/.62) as the benchmark to adjust the physician service component of expenditures for outpatient services on the MediCal file. MediCal expenditures for all other outpatient services such as pharmaceuticals, lab, x-ray, and clinic were added without adjustment to this adjusted physician component, thereby completing the construction of the CASR-OUT numerator. The resultant CASRs-OUT were applied to the total inpatient cost figures above to estimate total outpatient costs by condition and age (TCPREV).

Long-Term Care Costs

We made the conservative assumption that all costs of long-term care for the conditions of interest such as care in skilled nursing and intermediate care facilities were borne by MediCal, and that expenditures for such care were at cost.[e] Condition- and age-specific, long-term care costs were, therefore, adopted directly from the MediCal file, except for the costs of long-term care in the state' s seven developmental centers for those with Down syndrome and cerebral palsy. For these two conditions, estimates of costs of care in developmental centers were constructed from data on enrollment in these centers and overall budget data from the California Department of Developmental Services (DDS), as discussed below.

Long-term care in developmental centers — MediCal is virtually the sole source of funding for long-term care in the seven DDS-administered developmental centers in California. Had recording of diagnostic information been complete on MediCal claims, any claim for an individual with a birth defect of interest receiving care in developmental centers would have appeared on the MediCal file. However, as discussed in more detail below, diagnostic reporting for these centers on the MediCal claims file was inadequate. For two conditions (Down syndrome and cerebral palsy), we were able to obtain more reliable data on enrollment in these centers from our DDS file.[f] We, therefore, built a cost estimate according to Equation 2-5 based on DDS enrollment and budget data for these two conditions, as discussed below. Comprehensive enrollment data for the other birth defect categories were not available on the DDS file.[g] We, therefore, conservatively estimated long-term care costs for these other conditions based on unadjusted MediCal tape-to-tape claims data.

---

[e]A minor portion of long-term care in facilities for non-MediCal eligible clients is purchased by the California DDS. A small fraction of the costs of purchased developmental services reported in Chapter 5 for four birth defect categories, therefore, includes additional care in intermediate care and skilled nursing facilities for those born with these birth defects.

[f]See Appendix 2 for a description of the DDS data file.

[g]As discussed in Chapter 5, it is unlikely that enrollment data reported on the DDS were comprehensive for Down syndrome, as well. However, because Down syndrome is a significant underlying etiology for mental retardation, a qualifying condition for services in the DDS, reporting was likely to be more comprehensive for this condition on the DDS file than for other birth defect categories.

Expenditures of $487 million were made for California' s seven developmental centers in fiscal year 1988-1989. As noted above, the DDS was reimbursed for the "lion' s" share of funding for these developmental centers ($452 million) from MediCal.[h] Of the 6,739 clients in these centers in 1988-1989, we estimated from our DDS file that 35.2% (2,375) had cerebral palsy and 4.2% (280) had Down syndrome. On our MediCal file, however, claims from the developmental centers were recorded for only 175 clients with cerebral palsy and sixteen with Down syndrome. These figures reflect approximately 7.4% and 5.7%, respectively, of our expectation, given the above enrollment figures on the DDS file. A detailed investigation by analysts at Systemetrics, a private firm that maintains and distributes the MediCal tape-to-tape file, revealed that the diagnostic information on claims for these developmental centers were inadequate.[i] We, therefore, made an estimate of services provided by these centers for people with these two conditions based on Equation 2-5 using enrollment figures from the DDS file and the overall $487 million budget for these centers.

We estimated the proportion of those with Down syndrome and cerebral palsy less than age eighteen and more than age eighteen residing in the seven developmental centers in 1988 (p_i) by dividing the prevalence estimates (Table 3-4) by the enrollment estimates in these age categories from the DDS file. We applied these percentages to the estimates of survivors by age (S_i) to estimate the number in each cohort residing in developmental centers by age. This age-specific number was multiplied by $72,266, the average cost per capita of residing in these centers in 1988 ($PCAFF_i$), to estimate

---

[h]Budget figures are from the governor' s budget, California DDS.

[i]From the special analysis performed for the authors by Systemetrics, there were $345 million in total claims listed on the MediCal file for these developmental centers (compared to the $452 million expended by MediCal according to published budget figures). This discrepancy, however, only explains a part of the relatively small number of claims for people with cerebral palsy and Down syndrome. The analysis by Systemetrics also revealed that the most frequent diagnosis on claims from these centers was a missing diagnosis (15.5% of all claims) and that diagnoses for other claims were largely codes for acute conditions rather than the chronic problems for which these clients were admitted. Our selection criteria, in other words, were inadequate for flagging people with conditions of interest receiving care in the state' s developmental centers.

total costs at each age by condition. At a 5% discount rate, estimated total discounted costs in these developmental centers were $10.5 million for the cohort born in 1988 with Down syndrome and $66.4 million for those born with cerebral palsy (Table 4-3).

Even though the costs of long-term care in developmental centers for the other conditions were taken from the MediCal claims file, these figures by age and birth defect were enhanced by 7.4% of the developmental center' s budget that came from the DDS and did not appear on the MediCal file.

Other Medical Costs

Shriners—Two Shriners' hospitals in California provide inpatient and outpatient care to children with certain of the conditions of interest (i.e., spina bifida, missing limbs, and cerebral palsy), but data from these services do not appear on the OSHPD or MediCal data sets because these hospitals do not submit complete discharge abstracts. Condition- and age-specific expenditures for Shriners' services were estimated based on 1990 accounting data from Shriners. The San Francisco Shriners Hospital reportedly followed 6,037 children in 1991, of whom 779 (12.9%) had a diagnosis of cerebral palsy, 192 (3.2%) had spina bifida, and 82 (1.4%) had limb reductions. These percentages were applied to the $11 million total budget of that institution, which is less than a 10% offset for the estimated number of Mexican nationals in their patient population. Because the Los Angeles hospital was unable to provide such detailed data, we applied the percentages from San Francisco to the $12.5 million budget of the Los Angeles facility. These costs were allocated among age groups based on the estimated age distribution of prevalent cases in the California population.

Estimating Incremental Medical Costs

Per-capita inpatient and outpatient medical expenditures for the average person in the United States were obtained from the 1987 National Medical Care Expenditure Survey to estimate incremental medical costs. Computations for the same age categories as in the analysis of OSHPD and MediCal files were generated by the staff of the Center for General Health Services Intramural Research at the Agency for Health Care Policy and Research. These 1987 figures were adjusted to reflect 1988 medical costs based on the change in the medical care component of the Consumer Price Index between 1987 and 1988. Because the National Medical Care Expenditure Survey likely included persons with birth defects, we might have slightly overestimated the medical costs associated with defect-free survival. These population averages were subtracted from the gross costs above to estimate incremental costs. When the average per-capita costs exceeded the estimated cost for persons with a specific birth defect in any age category, the incremental costs were set equal to zero. In other words, we assumed that medical costs for people with a birth defect do not fall below the average age-specific per-capita medical costs of the noninstitutionalized population.

Results

Our estimates of gross per-capita medical costs by condition and age are reported in Table 4-2, as well as average per-capita medical costs among the U.S. population (bottom row). The difference between each condition entry and the corresponding average entry equals age-specific per-capita incremental medical costs ($PCPREV_i$). It is evident that the medical costs associated with most of these conditions are highly concentrated in the first few years of life, after which there is a precipitous drop. Substantial medical costs persist into adulthood, however, for several of the heart defects and for chronic conditions such as spina bifida, Down syndrome, and cerebral palsy. Large per-capita medical costs for cerebral palsy and Down syndrome in the 18+ age group reflect particularly large long-term care costs.

Final cohort estimates of direct medical costs of each condition (TC) were generated by multiplying the above per-capita costs by estimates of the cohort (S_i) (Equation 2-3) and appropriately discounting (Equation 2-1). These total cost estimates, broken down by inpatient, outpatient, and long-term care components, are reported in Table 4-3 at discount rates of 2%, 5%, and 10%, respectively.

Inpatient costs associated with the acute phase of illness tend to dominate medical care costs in the first year for the birth defects listed in quadrant I of Table 2-2 and for heart defects. For chronic conditions that persist into adulthood such as Down syndrome,

Table 4-2. Per-capita medical costs (a) by condition and age, and average United States per-capita medical cost (b), 1988 ($)

Condition	Age group			
	Zero to one	Two to four	Five to seventeen	Eighteen plus
Spina bifida	20,658	9,064	8,022	2,547
Truncus arteriosus	98,674	63,302	4,371	3,121
Transposition/DORV	34,192	9,590	1,865	1,059
Tetralogy of Fallot	42,958	11,511	3,607	760
Single ventricle	34,692	9,552	7,815	6,117
Cleft lip or palate	6,794	1,230	917	863
TE fistula	27,964	--	--	--
Atresia, small intestine	21,099	--	--	--
Colorectal atresia	15,349	2,557	248	--
Renal agenesis	10,654	1,261	646	550
Urinary obstruction	7,751	--	--	--
Upper-limp reduction	5,457	400	277	170
Lower-limp reduction	7,220	738	1,085	2,121
Diaphragmatic hernia	27,131	--	--	--
Gastroschisis	26,811	--	--	--
Omphalocele	20,461	--	--	--
Down syndrome (c)	16,560	3,387	1,355	4,573
Cerebral palsy (c)	9,861	5,981	6,955	11,752
Average United States cost	2,585	496	618	1,443

(a) Cost estimates are based on adjustments to the OSHPD and MediCal files, as discussed in the text.

(b) Figures are taken from the 1987 National Medical Expenditure Survey, adjusted to 1988 medical care prices.

(c) Estimates of long-term care costs in developmental centers for Down syndrome and cerebral palsy were calculated from California Department of Developmental Services budget and enrollment figures, as discussed in the text. The above per-capita entries for these two conditions include long-term care costs such as Down syndrome, less than age eighteen, $116, more than age eighteen, $2,478; cerebral palsy, less than age eighteen, $2,074, more than age eighteen, $8,663.

cerebral palsy, spina bifida, and limb reductions, the ratio of inpatient to outpatient costs tends to be lower. Because incremental medical care costs persist throughout adulthood for these conditions, they also are more heavily discounted than costs associated with conditions in which treatment is concentrated during the first two years of life. For this reason as well, the ratio of costs for conditions with concentrated early treatment to costs for conditions in which treatment is generally more spread out over the life span increases with the discount rate.

The total costs of medical care were highest for cerebral palsy, Down syndrome, spina bifida, and conotruncal heart defects. High costs for cerebral palsy and Down syndrome were partly driven by high incidence (Table 3-1), although the large medical costs associated with these two conditions were also driven more than the others by particularly large long-term care costs, reflecting long-term disabilities.

Average lifetime medical costs per case were highest for spina bifida ($99,000), conotruncal heart defects such as truncus arteriosus ($209,000), tetralogy of Fallot ($109,000), and single ventricle ($99,000), and cerebral palsy ($142,000).[j] Such costs were lowest for upper-limb reduction ($5,000). The denominator for these reported average lifetime medical costs per case is the size of the cohort at birth with each defect, including those who die within a few days of birth. Average medical costs were significantly larger, of course, for those who survived the neonatal period. A summary breakdown of total medical costs and cost per case by discount rate is provided in Table 4-4.

Our Estimates in Relation to Earlier Work

Prior to our study, there have been remarkably few studies undertaken of the lifetime medical costs associated with specific birth defects. One relatively recent study conducted in North Carolina on the cost effectiveness of screening for spina bifida provided medical cost estimates based on individual reviews of clinical records for 103 spina bifida victims in that state.[3] Despite differences in methodology between that study and our estimates, we made certain adjustments to construct a comparison between the two. The results

---

[j]All dollar figures in parentheses are provided at a 5% discount rate.

Table 4-3. Summary gross and net medical costs of birth defects in California by condition and type of service ($1,000s, 1988)

Condition	Gross inpatient	Inpatient as (%) of total	Gross outpatient	Outpatient as (%) of total	Long-term care	Long-term care as (%) of total	Gross total	Net total (a)
Spina bifida	15,545	(60.3)	9,806	(38.0)	427	(1.7)	25,778	22,402
Truncus arteriosus	9,343	(75.7)	2,934	(23.8)	72	(0.6)	12,349	11,784
Transposition/DORV	16,422	(76.4)	5,071	(23.6)	--	...	21,493	18,220
Tetralogy of Fallot	17,286	(75.9)	5,434	(23.9)	63	(0.3)	22,783	20,279
Single ventricle	5,795	(76.8)	1,736	(23.0)	12	(0.2)	7,543	6,754
Cleft lip or palate	16,061	(63.5)	9,108	(36.0)	144	(0.6)	25,312	10,639
TE fistula	6,376	(85.8)	1,054	(14.2)	--	...	7,430	6,743
Atresia, small intestine	6,423	(81.5)	1,462	(18.5)	--	...	7,885	6,919
Colorectal atresia	6,159	(77.8)	1,756	(22.2)	3	...	7,918	6,267
Renal agenesis	2,789	(63.6)	1,586	(36.2)	11	(0.3)	4,386	2,707
Urinary obstruction	5,903	(77.6)	1,682	(22.1)	23	(0.3)	7,608	5,072
Upper-limb reduction	1,574	(52.1)	1,441	(47.7)	7	(0.2)	3,022	1,220
Lower-limb reduction	1,906	(49.7)	1,873	(48.9)	55	(1.4)	3,834	1,814
Diaphragmatic hernia	6,122	(80.6)	1,478	(19.4)	--	...	7,600	6,876

Condition	Gross inpatient	Inpatient as (%) of total	Gross outpatient	Outpatient as (%) of total	Long-term care	Long-term care as (%) of total	Gross total	Net total (a)
Gastroschisis	5,502	(83.2)	1,107	(16.8)	--	..	6,609	5,972
Omphalocele	2,761	(83.2)	556	(16.8)	--	..	3,317	3,053
Down syndrome	20,686	(51.0)	9,396	(23.2)	10,460	(25.8)	40,542	30,528
Cerebral palsy	20,631	(19.7)	17,872	(17.0)	66,431	(63.3)	104,934	93,306

Note: Estimates beyond the first year of life are discounted at 5% back to age zero. Estimates are for care through the second year of life for conditions listed in quadrant I of Table 2-2, with the exception of colorectal atresia, for which estimates are through age seventeen. Congenital urinary tract obstruction may be associated with medical costs beyond the second year, but data limitations prevented estimation of such costs. For conditions listed in other quadrants of Table 2-2, estimates reflect costs through age sixty-five.

(a) Net costs equal gross costs minus the average cost of inpatient and outpatient medical care in the US population (see text).

84   The Cost of Birth Defects

Table 4-4. Summary net (a) medical costs of birth defects in
California by condition and discount rate ($1,000s, 1988)

Condition	Total cost by discount rate			Cost per case by discount rate		
	2%	5%	10%	2%	5%	10%
Spina bifida	28,851	22,402	17,027	128	99	75
Truncus arteriosus	12,855	11,784	10,809	228	209	192
Transposition/DORV	19,228	18,220	16,973	73	69	65
Tetralogy of Fallot	21,963	20,279	18,302	118	109	98
Single ventricle	9,410	6,754	5,131	138	99	75
Cleft lip or palate	11,540	10,639	9,597	12	11	10
TE fistula	6,826	6,743	6,615	44	44	43
Atresia, small intestine	7,013	6,919	6,773	35	35	34
Colorectal atresia	6,419	6,267	6,043	27	26	25
Renal agenesis	2,749	2,707	2,649	12	12	12
Urinary obstruction	5,136	5,071	4,971	9	9	9
Upper-limb reduction	1,236	1,220	1,195	5	5	5
Lower-limb reduction	2,783	1,814	1,304	24	16	11
Diaphragmatic hernia	6,935	6,876	6,784	35	35	34
Gastroschisis	6,051	5,972	5,851	44	44	43
Omphalocele	3,089	3,053	2,997	30	30	29
Down syndrome	48,236	30,528	21,475	86	55	39
Cerebral palsy	184,072	93,306	46,847	280	142	71

(a) Net costs equal gross costs minus the average cost of inpatient and outpatient medical care in the United States population (see text).

are reported in Table 4-5.

Lipscomb[4] made separate age-specific estimates for three locations of lesions in the open spina bifida victim: thoracic/high lumbar, low lumbar, and sacral. We constructed a weighted average of these three locations based upon weights provided by Lipscomb and tallied the medical costs reported in the North Carolina study for the same age categories as we report in Table 4-2. These are the figures

Table 4-5. Comparison of medical cost estimates per person with spina bifida by age group in two studies

Study	Age group			
	Zero to one	Two to four	Five to seventeen	Eighteen plus
Waitzman, Scheffler, and Romano (a)				
California, 1988	20,658	9,064	8,022	2,547
United States, 1988	18,729	8,218	7,273	2,309
Lipscomb (b)				
North Carolina, 1985	14,076	7,867	4,866	1,837
North Carolina, 1988	17,167	9,602	5,938	2,242

(a) California estimates are from Table 4-2, spina bifida entries. United States estimates are the California estimates deflated by difference in the employee compensation index in California and the United States (see text).

(b) Lipscomb made separate estimates for three lesion locations. The North Carolina 1985 estimates reflect a weighting of these three locations, as discussed in the text. The North Carolina 1988 estimates are the North Carolina 1985 estimates adjusted for medical care inflation from the consumer price index, south region (urban).

reported for North Carolina in 1985 (Table 4-5). We made additional adjustments because of differences in medical care prices between California and North Carolina and between the base years of the studies: 1985 and 1988. We deflated our California estimates by the difference in the Employee Compensation Index between California and the nation in 1988 from the Bureau of Labor Statistics.[k] We also inflated the 1985 Lipscomb estimates to 1988 based on the increase in the medical care component of the Consumer Price Index, south region (urban). Any remaining price differences would be attributable to differences between North Carolina and the nation in 1988. Differences in medical practice patterns between the two states also could account for differences in final estimates.

---

[k]We used the Employee Compensation Index because inpatient and outpatient medical costs were adjusted to Medicare cost schedules, which tend to be below reimbursement from commercial insurance. The remaining difference in costs between California and the United States, as a whole, is likely to be related predominantly to differences in the cost of living.

Despite the significant methodological differences between the two studies, the adjusted age-specific medical costs reported in Table 4-5 (bold type) bear a striking resemblance to each other. Our results for the age zero to one group suggest that some of the medical care attributed by Lipscomb[5] to ages two to four, based on his relatively small sample, actually may have transpired earlier on average. Our significantly higher estimates for the age five to seventeen group also suggests that medical care for those born with spina bifida declined at a more gradual rate over the life span than suggested by the Lipscomb estimate. The fundamental congruence between the estimates in the two studies is striking, however, given the differences in the two studies' approaches.

A recent study on the cost of brain disorders included an estimate for the cost of cerebral palsy under the prevalence approach.[6] It is difficult to make direct comparisons from this study to our estimates because of differences in underlying methodology. The 1991 estimate of aggregate inpatient and outpatient medical care costs associated with treatment of cerebral palsy from this study was $367 million. The Lewin study did not calculate costs associated with long-term care. The corresponding estimate from our analysis adjusted to 1991 medical care prices and projected to the nation was $228 million at a 5% discount rate.

The substantial discrepancy between these two estimates are attributable primarily to the different impact of discounting between the two approaches but also to our attempt to isolate incremental costs. We discuss these and other differences with respect to the above study in more detail in Chapter 7. We believe that our focus on incremental costs and our use of actual financial records related to units of service for treatment of cerebral palsy (the Lewin-ICF study relied on average expenditures for all diseases) represent an improvement over the Lewin-ICF methodology. We encourage researchers to undertake additional estimates of the medical costs of this and other birth defects.

Endnotes to Chapter 4

1.Prospective Payment Commission. *Medicaid Hospital Payment: Congressional Report.* C-91-02; October 1, 1991.

2.Physician Payment Review Commission. *Physician Payment Under Medicaid.* Washington, DC: Author; 1991.

3.Lipscomb J. *Human capital, willingness-to-pay, and cost-effectiveness analysis of screening for birth defects in North Carolina.* Presented at the annual meeting of the American Economic Association; December 28, 1986; New Orleans, Louisiana.

4.Ibid.

5.Ibid.

6.National Foundation for Brain Research. *The Cost of Disorders of the Brain.* Washington, DC: Author; 1992.

Chapter 5

Nonmedical Direct Costs of Birth Defects: Developmental Services and Special Education

Introduction

Those born with certain birth defects often experience developmental problems and disabilities that are not fully correctable through medical care. Special resources for functioning on a daily basis, participating in normal activities, and coping with situations encountered in everyday life are often required. For birth defects listed outside of quadrant I of Table 2-2, such requirements were expected to be the rule rather than the exception. Mental retardation of varying severity is a trademark of Down syndrome but also affects significant numbers of those with spina bifida and cerebral palsy. Orthopedic impairments associated with limb reductions, spina bifida, and cerebral palsy often require special equipment and services in order to restore function, as do neurological impairments associated with spina bifida and cerebral palsy.

In this chapter, we focus on the costs associated with two major categories of nonmedical direct services for those with birth defects listed outside of quadrant I of Table 2-2: (a) developmental services and (b) special education. These two categories of service are similar to each other; that is, large, publicly financed, and administered programs generally are devoted to their provision. In California, the

Department of Developmental Services (DDS) and the Department of Education manage these programs. The estimates we provide are for the publicly provided portion of these services only, although some comparable services are undoubtedly purchased privately.

We do not estimate the full component of nonmedical direct services such as the devotion of family members' time and other resources, which may be substantial for children born with certain birth defects. To the extent that publicly provided respite and day program services purchased by the DDS (see below) substitute for usual commitments from family members, however, that portion is incorporated into our estimates.

Direct Costs of Developmental Services

What are Developmental Services?

The California DDS is authorized under the Lanterman Developmental Disabilities Services Act (hereafter "the Act") of 1977 to administer the Developmental Disabilities Service Delivery System in California. Under the Act, people are eligible for developmental services if they have one or more of four specific qualifying disabilities: (a) mental retardation, (b) cerebral palsy or like dysfunction, (c) epilepsy, or (d) autism. People with other disabilities can qualify under a general fifth category if their disability is similar to mental retardation or requires services similar to those required by the mentally retarded.

The DDS serves an annual client base in California of approximately 100,000. A client typically makes initial contact with the DDS through one of twenty-one private, nonprofit "regional centers" in the state. A major responsibility of the regional center is to place clients in the appropriate residential setting. While close to 60% of the DDS clients lived in their own homes in 1988, approximately 22% and 6% lived in community care facilities and skilled nursing/intermediate care health facilities, respectively. In addition, approximately 7% were placed in one of the state' s seven residential "developmental centers." The developmental centers are administered by the DDS but receive most of their funding through MediCal. The costs associated with long-term care for clients with birth defects of interest in these centers were incorporated in the medical cost estimates presented in Chapter 4.

A variety of developmental services is provided directly from DDS personnel, whereas others are purchased by the DDS. Direct services include information and referral, intake, diagnosis and evaluation, counseling, assessment, program planning, and case management. Purchased services fall into in five general categories:

1. Out-of-home. For clients who do not live in their own home, DDS purchases services in licensed community care facilities (CCF) or in a variety of health institutions such as intermediate care facilities (ICF) and skilled nursing facilities (SNF) for non-MediCal eligible clients

2. Day program. Nursery programs, family day care programs, and other day care facilities for adults and children with developmental disabilities

3. Medical services. Inpatient and outpatient care, pharmaceuticals, laboratory tests, and appliances

4. Camps (day, residential, and traveling) and respite (licensed vocational nurses, respite care facilities, home health agencies and aides, homemakers and homemaker programs)

5. Other services (nonmedical professionals, interpreters, driver training, attorneys, prevention services, transportation, independent living skills, sensory motor programs not provided in residential settings, as well as others).

General Budget for Developmental Services

The approximately $1 billion annual budget for the DDS in fiscal year 1988-1989 was roughly divided equally between the operating budget for the seven developmental centers and the regional centers' activities of direct and purchased client services. As noted above, DDS is reimbursed for nearly all of the operating budget for the developmental centers by MediCal and other public funds. Of the $460 million allocated to the activities of the regional centers, approximately $333 million (72.5%) was devoted to purchase of services, whereas the remaining $127 million was allocated to direct operations. Most purchases of services were for out-of-home care (39%), other services (29%), and day programs (25%). The other categories (respite/camps and medical care) made up 5% and 2% of purchased services, respectively.

General Method for Calculating Developmental Services Costs

The general method we adopted for calculating the developmental service costs of birth defects is summarized by Equation 2-4 and is reprinted here as Equation 5-1:

$$TC_i = S_i \times p_i \times PCAFF_i, \qquad\qquad [5\text{-}1]$$

where TC_i is the total cost of developmental services for a birth defect at age i, S_i is the estimated number of survivors with a specific birth defect at age i from the 1988 birth cohort, p_i is the proportion of the prevalent population with the defect at age i that receives developmental services, and $PCAFF_i$ is the per-capita cost among this "affected" prevalent population at age i. Estimates of these age-specific total costs for those receiving services are discounted and summed according to Equation 2-1 to arrive at the final costs of developmental services by condition.

As we stressed in our discussion of general methodology in Chapter 2, we have taken care in our analysis to estimate only incremental costs, that is, costs above and beyond what a child born without congenital anomalies would incur. In the case of developmental services costs, however, we treated the cost estimates from our DDS data as incremental costs because the probability of receiving services through DDS among the general population in California for conditions other than for birth defects of interest was very small, in fact, well below 1%.

Because we relied on DDS data for population and cost estimates, as discussed below, there is a natural tripartite division to the estimation of the cost of developmental services corresponding to the three general budget categories mentioned above: (a) purchase of services, (b) direct provision of services, and (c) services delivered through the state' s seven developmental centers. Cost estimates for the first two categories are provided below. Services delivered in developmental centers for those with birth defects were incorporated into the estimates of long-term care costs in Chapter 4.

We used client-specific DDS data on purchases of services (by service category) in fiscal year 1988-1989 to estimate this component of developmental costs. Care was taken not to double-count services incorporated into other parts of the study. For example, we made an estimate of the total cost of medical care by birth defect in Chapter

4; thus, we excluded DDS-purchased medical care in calculating the cost of purchased developmental services for those with birth defects. Client-specific cost data were unavailable on direct provision of services. We, therefore, added a direct service component to purchase of services based on the percentage of the 1988-1989 DDS budget devoted to direct operating expenses.

Data

Population and purchase of developmental services estimates by birth defect category were made from a specially created 10% randomly selected subfile of clients provided through DDS. The subfile contained client-specific diagnostic and evaluative information from DDS' Client Development Evaluation Report (CDER) merged with financial data on purchases of services from the DDS "masterfile" for 9,125 clients in fiscal year 1988-1989.

In addition to listing a DDS client' s qualifying condition(s) such as mental retardation, cerebral palsy, autism, epilepsy, or "other like mental retardation," the CDER report, beginning in 1984, listed up to two underlying etiologies (ICD-9 codes) for each qualifying condition. Furthermore, the CDER report recorded up to five medical conditions (ICD-9 codes) that contribute significantly to the client' s developmental needs, even if the condition was not an underlying etiology for a qualifying condition. In order to estimate the population with birth defects of interest that receive DDS services, we selected all of those with the qualifying condition of cerebral palsy and like dysfunction (adjusted to those with cerebral palsy only as discussed below), as well as anyone with the ICD-9 code of a birth defect of interest recorded as any underlying etiology or contributing medical condition.

Even though a minimum of one update is made annually to the CDER report, it is unlikely that all underlying etiologies (ICD-9 codes) for qualifying conditions were recorded retroactive to their initial integration into the CDER report in 1984 for clients eligible before 1984. It is, therefore, likely that we underestimated the number of people with birth defects of interest receiving DDS services.

The qualifying condition for cerebral palsy was modified in 1986 to include "like dysfunction." Based on a DDS report indicating that expansion of the qualifying criterion was responsible for an increase of 2% in the proportion of the DDS client base with cerebral palsy between 1985 and 1990,[1] we accordingly adjusted downward the reported number of those with "cerebral palsy and like dysfunction" to estimate those strictly with cerebral palsy. Based on this adjustment, there were 2,083 respondents on the DDS file with cerebral palsy. From the recorded ICD-9 codes for underlying etiologies and contributing medical conditions, there were 631 clients with Down syndrome, 36 with spina bifida, and 21 with cleft lip or palate.[a] These population estimates from our 10% file were multiplied by ten to make a point estimate of the full DDS population (AFFPOP) in California with conditions of interest in 1988.

The above population estimates, stratified by the four age categories used for overall prevalence estimates provided in Table 3-4, were divided by those prevalence (PREVPOP$_i$) figures to estimate the proportion of each cohort by age and condition in California who were DDS clients in 1988 (p$_i$). Estimates of these proportions are provided in Table 5-1. By age five, our data indicated that approximately 90% of those with cerebral palsy in the state received developmental services through DDS. Given that mental retardation is a qualifying condition for eligibility for DDS services, it is not surprising that approximately 75% of those with Down syndrome between the ages of zero to four are estimated to receive such services. The decline in this percentage in older age groups likely reflects underreporting due to the absence of underlying etiologies (ICD-9 codes) on CDER reports prior to 1984 (see above), as well as higher mortality at younger ages among those with the most severe Down syndrome.

We made developmental services cost estimates only for conditions and age groups in which more than 1% of the population with the condition were estimated to receive services. Developmental service cost estimates for cleft lip or palate were, therefore, made only through age four.

According to the general methodology summarized in Equation 5-1, we multiplied the condition- and age-specific proportions (p$_i$) in Table 5-1 by our estimates of the cohort alive at each age (S$_i$) to

---

[a]Several clients had other birth defects of interest, but there were not sufficient numbers with any of these other conditions to make reliable cost estimates.

Table 5-1. Proportion receiving developmental services from the California Department of Developmental Services, 1988-1989 (FY), by condition and age

Condition	Age group			
	Zero to one	Two to four	Five to seventeen	Eighteen plus
Spina bifida	.08	.12	.10	.02
Cleft lip or palate	.02	.03	(a)	(a)
Down syndrome	.76	.73	.47	.35
Cerebral palsy	.61	.76	.87	.66

Note: These figures are based upon enrollment data from the California Department of Developmental Services' file divided by prevalence estimates by corresponding age group in Table 3-4.

(a) Less than .01.

estimate the number of people in the cohort receiving developmental services at each age by condition. This cohort figure was multiplied by the per-capita purchases of nonmedical services on the DDS file by condition and age ($PCAFF_i$) provided in Table 5-2 to estimate condition- and age-specific total costs (TC_i) of purchased developmental services. This figure was enhanced by our estimate of direct services provided per dollar of purchased services, as discussed earlier. Estimates of total developmental costs for each condition after appropriate discounting and summing of the above age-specific costs are provided in Table 5-3.

Results

The total estimated cost of developmental services for those with Down syndrome, discounted at 5%, was $12 million, approximately two thirds of the total lifetime inpatient medical costs for that condition (Table 4-3). The corresponding total developmental services cost for those with cerebral palsy was $27.5 million, approximately 33% higher than the $20.6 million in lifetime inpatient costs associated with the disease. Total estimated DDS expenditures for clients with spina bifida and cleft lip or palate were far lower than for the other two conditions ($225,000 and $371,000, respectively). Per-capita costs for those with spina bifida are more than twice that

Table 5-2. Total and per-capita purchases of developmental services
($) by condition and age group, 1988-1989 (FY)

Condition	Age group		
	Zero to four	Five to seventeen	Eighteen plus
Spina bifida			
Total	5,456	20,010	18,952
Medical	175	16,996	2,114
Net	5,281	3,014	16,838
Net/capita	587	188	1,531
Total/capita	606	1,250	1,723
Cleft lip or palate			
Total	32,568		
Medical	6,278		
Net	26,290		
Net/capita	2,390	(a)	(a)
Total/capita	2,691		
Down syndrome			
Total	323,405	171,572	1,100,287
Medical	44,093	19,647	4,641
Net	279,309	151,925	1,095,646
Net/capita	1,643	821	3,970
Total/capita	1,902	927	3,987
Cerebral palsy			
Total	417,125	1,493,044	4,940,364
Medical	131,196	380,649	255,248
Net	285,929	1,112,395	4,685,116
Net/capita	973	1,460	3,797
Total/capita	1,419	1,959	4,004

Note: Cost figures are purchases of services from the California Department of Developmental Services (DDS) 10%
file. Net figures are totals minus medical purchases. Per-capita figures reflect totals divided by the number of eligible
clients by age and condition from the DDS file. Net per-capita figures are used to estimate the purchase of service
component of developmental services' costs, whereas total per capital figures are used to estimate the cost of services
directly provided by DDS personnel (see text).

(a) Cost of developmental services for those with cleft lip or palate are restricted to those under age four because less
than 1% of those more than four are estimated to receive developmental services.

for cleft lip or palate, but total costs for cleft lip or palate are higher
because of the higher incidence of the disease.

Direct Costs of Special Education

In this section, estimates are provided of the cost of special
education services for students with the conditions of interest listed

Table 5-3. Total and per-capita costs of developmental services by condition in California, 1988-1989 (FY)

Condition	Total cost by discount rate ($000s)			Cost per case (a) by discount rate ($)		
	2%	5%	10%	2%	5%	10%
Spina bifida	370	225	138	1,636	993	610
Cleft lip or palate	395	371	338	418	394	358
Down syndrome	22,914	12,004	6,466	41,085	21,524	11,594
Cerebral palsy	57,903	27,525	12,312	88,132	41,895	18,739

Note: Developmental services include the purchase and direct provision of nonmedical services by the California Department of Developmental Services (DDS) based on estimates from the DDS 10% file. (See text and Appendix 2 for a fuller description of such services and the data file.) Even though all conditions listed in quadrants II and IV of Table 2-2 would be expected to generate requirements for such services above the average for the general population, restrictions on eligibility for DDS services and limitations of the data file permitted estimation of such costs for these four conditions only (see text).

(a) Cost-per-case estimates are total cost estimates divided by the number of individuals born with each condition in 1988 in California.

in quadrants II and IV of Table 2-2, except renal agenesis/dysgenesis. Even though it is likely that children born with renal agenesis/dysgenesis receive more special education services, on average, than the child without birth defects, our data were not sufficiently rich to estimate the extent of such services.

Under the Individuals with Disabilities Education Act (IDEA) (formerly the Education for All Handicapped Children Act), public schools are required to identify children from birth to age twenty-one with disabilities, evaluate their needs, and provide services tailored to those needs necessary for participation in school.[2] Enrollment in special education programs steadily increased during the 1980s to more than 4.6 million children in the 1988-1989 school year.[3] Approximately 10% of the school-age population received some special education services during that year.

General Method

Studies on the cost of special education generally have taken one of two approaches. One approach is the expenditure method, under which aggregate program budgets at the district level, including an aliquot portion of indirect costs, are divided by the number of children served by the program to estimate per-pupil costs. The major difficulties encountered with this approach are that district expenditures often are not broken down at the program level, and districts often differ in terms of special education accounting methods.[4] Under the second resource allocation method, costs are built up from individual service components provided to children in each program. It is often difficult, however, to determine the precise direct and indirect services that special education students receive.[5,6]

Two major studies of the resource allocation approach are those sponsored by Rand[7] and Decision Resources Corporation.[8] Our analysis represents an intermediate approach that recognizes the major finding in the Rand and Decision Resources Corporation studies that federal handicap and school placement categories are important predictors of variation in the costs of special education. The approach we undertook, however, utilizes aggregate categorical cost and enrollment data by school district in California to estimate, through regression analysis, the average cost associated with each placement and handicap category. These estimates, coupled with data on the distribution of students with underlying conditions of interest by relevant category, yielded estimates of cost by condition.

This approach to the calculation of special education costs for students with birth defects represents an extension beyond previous research that accepted national cost estimates as relevant to a particular state or assumed that students with an underlying condition were exclusively in one handicap category. The methodology is outlined in more detail below.

Specific Method

The specific method of estimating the cost of special education was based on Equation 2-4, reprinted as Equation 5-1 above. Specific refinements were incorporated into our methodology, however, to account for evidence in the cost of special education literature, suggesting that costs are sensitive to the federal handicap category and school placement settings.[9,10]

Students with disabilities requiring special education fit into one of eleven federal handicap categories, ranging from specific problems such as "deaf" and "blind" to more general classifications such as "mentally retarded," "orthopedically impaired," and "multiply handicapped." In addition, depending upon the severity of one's disability, a student is placed into one of four placement settings in California, which are not atypical of the placement settings in other states. These settings are regular classrooms with designated services, resource room or specialist, special day classes, or special school.

Because of the wide variation in resources provided to special education students, depending on their disability and school placement,[11,12] we incorporated refinements into our methodology to consider variation for special education students born with birth defects. The per-capita cost estimate of special education among those with each birth defect requiring such services (PCAFF) was constructed as a weighted sum of per-capita special education costs for each federal handicap category:

$$PCAFF = \Sigma_j \, fc_j \times PCFC_j, \qquad\qquad [5\text{-}2]$$

where fc_j equals the proportion of the affected population (those with the birth defect requiring special education) in the jth federal handicap category (j = 1-11), and $PCFC_j$ is an estimate of per-capita special education costs in this jth category. In order to reflect differences in cost by placement setting, these per-capita federal handicap category costs were broken down further and estimated as the weighted sum of the per-capita cost by placement setting:

$$PCFC_j = \Sigma_k \, PCFC_{jk} \times CALPROP_{jk}, \qquad\qquad [5\text{-}3]$$

where $PCFC_{jk}$ is an estimate of the per-capita cost of special education for the jth federal handicap category in the kth placement setting (k = 1-4), and $CALPROP_{jk}$ is the proportion of California special education students in the jth federal handicap category and kth placement setting.[b] Substituting Equation 5-3 for $PCFC_j$ in Equation 5-2 and then substituting this modified Equation 5-2 for PCAFF in Equation 5-1 yields a modified equation for the total cost of special education for each birth defect:

---

[b]Students with birth defects were assumed to be distributed across placement settings according to the average among special education students in California in the same federal handicap category.

$$TC = S \times p \times (\Sigma_j fc_j \times (\Sigma_k PCFC_{jk} \times CALPROP_{jk})). \qquad [5\text{-}4]$$

Our procedure for estimating each component of this equation is provided below.

Linking Method to Data

Proportion receiving special education (p) — Estimates of the proportion of students with underlying conditions of interest receiving special education (p_i) were made from the pooled 1985-1989 National Health Interview Survey (NHIS) based on whether parents indicated that their children aged five to seventeen "attended" or "needed" special education.[c,13,d]   (See Appendix 2 for a description of the NHIS sample.)

All respondents to the NHIS were queried with respect to activity limitations because of their health. Parents of children between the ages of five and seventeen were asked about the specific limitations of their children with respect to school attendance if they indicate that their children have activity limitations. A potential drawback to these estimates from the NHIS is that the activity limitation question acted as a gatekeeper to the specific question regarding school attendance. Some children receiving special education (particularly those in regular education settings), however, may not be considered by their parents to have activity limitations. In addition, parents may not even be aware that their children receive special education

---

[c]The NHIS has been similarly used to estimate the proportion of children born with low birthweight requiring special education.

[d]The estimate of this proportion for those with Down syndrome was based on the overall proportion requiring special education among those listed with congenital mental retardation. Similarly, estimates for the heart conditions reflect the rate among all of those with congenital heart defects. From the SRI survey (Appendix 2), the distribution of students with Down syndrome across level of mental retardation categories revealed that those with Down syndrome were more concentrated among those with severe and moderate mental retardation than the mentally retarded as a whole. This was similarly the case on the DDS file for those with Down syndrome receiving developmental services.

services.[e,14]   Our estimates of the percentages of students with certain birth defects receiving special education, therefore, may be too low, particularly for those who have the slightest impairments with respect to school attendance and performance.

Estimates from the NHIS sample indicate that 83% of school-age children with Down syndrome, 60% with cerebral palsy, 51% with spina bifida, 16% with cleft lip or palate, 25% with upper-limb reductions, 26% with lower-limb reductions, and 8% with congenital heart defects receive special education (Table 5-4). Aside from those attending or needing special education, a substantial proportion of the remainder for several of the conditions was unable to attend school because of their limitation: (a) an estimated 10% of those with congenital mental retardation, (b) an estimated 10% of those with cerebral palsy, and (c) an estimated 15% of those with spina bifida (Table 5-4).

Federal handicap category (fc)—We estimated the distribution of those with each birth defect requiring special education among federal handicap categories based on parental and school reports of disabling conditions and federal handicap categories from the National Longitudinal Transition Study of Special Education Students conducted by Stanford Research International (Stanford Research International survey). The Stanford Research International survey was a nationally representative random sample of the special education population conducted in 1985 with more than 8,000 respondents. The file contains separate parent, school record, and school district components in addition to others that can be linked by a respondent's identification number. Up to fourteen underlying disabilities/conditions from the parent questionnaire and up to seventeen disabilities/conditions from the school record abstract are provided on the file. Even though this information was not provided

---

[e]In other research on the cost of special education in which the NHIS has been used, it has been suggested that this type of underreporting on the NHIS is most likely for speech-impaired students who receive most of their education in regular education classroom settings. NHIS estimates of the proportion of the population receiving special education are approximately equal to the national estimates minus the speech impaired.

Except for a proportion of those with cleft lip and/or palate, speech impairment is unlikely to be the primary handicap category of those with underlying conditions.

The Cost of Birth Defects

Table 5-4. School limitations by condition (ages five to seventeen)

Condition	Total prevalence	Unable to attend (%)	Attends/needs special education (a) (%)	Limited in attendance (%)	No school limitation (%)
Spina bifida	68,049	10,766 (16)	34,610 (51)	15,160 (22)	7,514 (11)
Cleft lip or palate	280,234	--	45,153 (16)	--	235,081 (84)
Upper-limb reduction	47,051	--	11,776 (25)	--	20,019 (75)
Lower-limb reduction	45,654	--	11,776 (26)	--	26,358 (74)
Cerebral palsy	328,544	27,386 (08)	197,973 (60)	45,919 (16)	57,266 (17)
Congenital mental retardation (b)	568,259	61,270 (11)	473,456 (83)	--	33,532 (06)
Congenital heart defect (c)	123,987	--	9,530 (08)	9,706 (08)	82,492 (74)

Note: Weighted estimates based upon the National Health Interview Survey (NHIS), 1985-1989.

(a) Percentages in this column used to estimate the proportion receiving special education.

(b) Used to estimate proportion of those with Down syndrome receiving special education.

(c) Used to estimate proportion of those with conotruncal heart defects (truncus arteriosus, transposition/DORV, tetralogy of Fallot, and single ventricle) receiving special education.

from a checklist of conditions, in most instances a birth defect of interest was listed by both school and parent of the respondent when it was listed by one or the other. Birth defects also were listed among comorbidities as the primary reason for requiring special education services for the vast majority of cases in which a congenital condition was listed at all.

We assumed that the national distribution by federal category from the Stanford Research International survey applied, in general, to California.[f,15] Cleft lip or palate was not listed on the survey as an underlying condition. Several of those born with a cleft deformity probably received special education services related to associated comorbidities or were listed under more general disability categories on the survey. We, therefore, assumed that the distribution across placement and handicap categories for cleft lip or palate was the same as that for the overall special education population in California. The distribution of students with "amputation of a limb" was used as a proxy to estimate the distribution of those with upper- and lower-limb reductions.

The federal handicap category for each respondent was assigned in the Stanford Research International "combined data file" based on an algorithm developed by Stanford Research International that utilizes information on placement from the school district or from information on underlying disabilities in which district information was absent or otherwise inadequate. Table 5-5 provides the distribution of students among the eleven federal handicap categories by condition (fc_j) from the Stanford Research International "combined data file."[g] Not unexpectedly, those with Down syndrome were concentrated in the mentally retarded category, those with cerebral palsy were concentrated in the mental retardation, orthopedically impaired, and multiply handicapped categories, whereas the largest proportion of those with spina bifida and missing limb were in the orthopedically impaired category.

---

[f]State-specific estimates by the US Department of Education estimates of special education students by federal handicap category supported this assumption.

[g]The distribution reflects categories that contain at least 5% of all respondents with the underlying condition.

The Cost of Birth Defects

Table 5-5. Distribution of special education students by federal special handicap category by condition

Condition	Learning disabled	Orthopedically impaired	Mental retardation	Other health impaired	Multiply handicapped
Spina bifida	.38	.48	. .	. .	.14
Heart (a)	.18	. .	.60	.11	.11
Amputation of limb (b)	.23	.77	. .	. .	. .
Down syndrome	. .	. .	.95	. .	.05
Cerebral palsy	.17	.20	.43	. .	.17

Note: Based on Stanford Research International (SRI) Longitudinal Survey of special education studies. (See text for a description of data and methodology.)

(a) The distribution for heart problems is applied to all those with conotruncal heart defects (common truncus, transposition/DORV, tetralogy of Fallot, and single ventricle) estimated to receive special education.

(b) The distribution for amputation of limb is applied to those with congenital upper- or lower-limb reductions estimated to receive special education.

Per-capita cost by handicap and placement (PCFC$_{jk}$) —Per-capita special education cost by federal handicap category for each placement setting (PCFC$_{jk}$) was estimated from regressions that utilized California special education enrollment data merged to California expenditure data at the district level. District-level special education enrollment data for the 1988-1989 school year by age (zero to twenty-two), federal handicap category, and school placement category were obtained from the California State Department of Education, Special Education Division. District-level special education expenditure data by the four placement categories from the J-380 Annual Program Cost Data Report also were obtained from the School Business Services Division of the California State Department of Education. These cost data included direct costs, direct support costs, and indirect costs, as defined by the Department of Education. Direct costs include program-specific expenditures such as teachers' salaries and textbooks, as well as prorated expenditures for multiple-program and more generalized services. Direct support costs include costs of support services programs such as instructional media, instructional and school administration, pupil services, and transportation. These costs are distributed to specific activities by the Department of Education based upon direct documentation or various weighted allocation methods. A portion of other major support service programs (centralized data processing, plant maintenance, and plant operations) also are treated as direct support costs, whereas the remainder is allocated as indirect costs. District-level cost data on regionalized services, transportation, and assessment activities related to special education also were provided but not broken down into placement categories. These costs were distributed on a per-capita basis to placement category.

Regressions were estimated based on the following equation:

$$D_k = \alpha_k + \Sigma_j \beta_{jk} H_{jk} + \epsilon_k \qquad\qquad [5\text{-}5]$$

where D_k is total special education costs at the district level for the kth placement category (k = 1-4); α is an intercept term; H_{jk} is district-level enrollment in the jth federal handicap category (j = 1-11) in the kth placement category; $\beta_{jk} = PCFC_{jk}$ is the coefficient of interest indicating the increase in cost with an increase in enrollment of one student in handicap category j within placement setting k; and ϵ_k is an error term.[h] Enrollment and cost data were provided on 799 school districts (observations) in the state, but only districts that had positive enrollments in a placement category were included in any placement-specific regression.

Estimates of the costs per special education pupil by federal handicap and school placement categories ($PCFC_{jk}$) from the regressions are provided in Table 5-6. As with earlier studies, placement in nonpublic school (NPS) was generally the most costly, placement in special day classes (SPC) the next most costly, whereas placement in resource specialist (RSP) and designated instructional services (DIS) were the least costly settings. The estimate of the cost for a student in the "learning disabled" federal handicap category, for example, was $2,882 for DIS, $3,532 for RSP, $5,509 for SPC, and $21,548 for NPS.

The distribution of students among placements (CALPROP_jk)—The distribution of students across the j federal handicap categories and the k placement settings was estimated

---

[h]Because districts with larger enrollments have larger expenditures, weighted least squares regressions were conducted to adjust for heteroskedasticity.

Table 5-6. Regression results on the costs of special education in
California by placement category

Federal handicap category	Placement			
	Designated instructional services	Resource specialist	Special day classes	Nonpublic school
Speech impaired	2,320 (a)	3,197 (b)	7,198 (a)	
Other handicap	3,617	33,184 (a)	35,803 (a)	
Orthopedically impaired	9,778		14,941 (a)	
Visually handicapped	45,869 (a)		11,615 (a)	
Hard of hearing	23,267 (b)		8,990 (b)	
Learning disabled	2,882 (c)	3,532 (a)	5,509 (a)	21,548 (a)
Mentally retarded			12,904 (a)	21,285 (a)
Multiply handicapped			10,403 (a)	28,788 (a)
Emotionally disabled			14,324 (a)	19,084 (a)
Deaf			18,851 (a)	
Intercept	62,372 (a)	3,624	14,654 (c)	4,342
Adjusted R^2	.303	.864	.936	.862
N (districts)	551	767	627	271

(a) $p < .01$.

(b) $p < .05$.

(c) $p < .10$.

directly from the California Department of Education's special
education enrollment data. Nearly all of those in the learning
disabled category in California, for example, were in RSP (68%) or
SPD (29%). The estimated per-capita cost for the learning disabled
federal category, $PCFC_j$ (Equation 5-3), therefore, was heavily
weighted by these placements. Per-capita cost estimates by federal
handicap category ($PCFC_j$), after accounting for displacement of
regular education costs (see below), are given in Table 5-7.

Incremental Costs

Had they been born without birth defects, a portion of the birth cohorts for which we estimate costs would still require special education services, presumably at the rate of the general population. Furthermore, even within the special education setting, certain resources merely displace those that would have been utilized in any case in a regular education setting. Other resources, on the other hand, are a net of the usual costs of education. Both of these factors (the experience of the general population with respect to special education and the extent to which special education displaces regular education costs) were incorporated into our estimates in the manner discussed below, thus making incremental cost estimates.

Adjustment for displacement of regular education—The degree to which special education displaces regular education largely depends upon placement. Some placements such as nonpublic school (NPS) nearly displaces all regular education services for students in such settings. On the other hand, for those receiving designated instructional services in regular school settings, special education costs generally will be wholesale additions to regular education costs. In order to calculate incremental costs of special education over and above regular education costs, we subtracted a percentage of regular education costs, based upon the findings of the study by Moore et al.[16] on the extent to which each placement category, on average, displaces regular education.[i] Nearly all students in the mentally retarded federal handicap category in California, for example, are placed in SDC. Based on the above study, placement displaces 52% of regular education. The average cost per pupil for the mentally retarded category ($PCFC_j$) reported in Table 5-7, therefore, reflects

---

[i]Based on this study, special education did not displace any regular education in the designated instructional services and resource specialist placements, thereby making the special education costs for these placements in Table 5-7 fully incremental. However, 51% and 84% of regular education were displaced by SDC and NPS, respectively; thus, these percentages of regular education costs were subtracted from costs in these categories to estimate incremental special education costs.

the subtraction of 52% of the cost of regular education.[j] Regular education costs of $2,928 per pupil were figured based on summary figures from the J-380 expenditure spreadsheet provided by the Department of Education for fiscal year 1988-1989,[k] divided by regular education enrollment figures for grades K-12 from the state for the same year.

Age-specific, per-pupil costs by birth defect (PCAFF) were estimated according to Equation 5-2 by multiplying the federal handicap category distribution by birth defect (fc$_j$) in Table 5-5 by the corresponding per-pupil cost estimates by federal handicap category (PCFC$_i$) in Table 5-7 and summing these products. As an example, 95% of those with Down syndrome requiring special education were placed in the mentally retarded category, whereas 5% were multiply handicapped (Table 5-5). These percentages were multiplied by the estimated costs in Table 5-7 for mental retardation and multiple handicap placements, respectively, and then summed to arrive at $11,416, which is the estimate of the annual education cost for a student with Down syndrome requiring special education (PCAFF).[l] These annual per-pupil special education costs by birth defect

---

[j]This is a slight simplification. A small percentage (1.4%) of those in the mentally retarded category in California are placed in NPS, which displaces 84% of regular education. This distribution is reflected in the overall incremental cost for the mentally retarded category.

[k]These costs of regular education were taken from line 130, "Total, General Education."

[l]Our estimates for special education costs for several birth defect categories may be conservative. We have assumed that the cost by each birth defect category is the average of the federal handicap category across the four placements. However, evidence from the Stanford Research International survey indicated that those with birth defects were concentrated in more expensive placement settings than the average for the federal handicap categories in which they fell. Placement settings were provided on the Stanford Research International survey, and we assigned those with birth defects to placements on the survey based on the California procedure for assignment of a single setting to each respondent. There was greater concentration of those with birth defects (e.g., Down syndrome, cerebral palsy, and spina bifida, in particular) in more expensive placements such as nonpublic schools than the California average for the federal handicap categories in which they fell. We did not use the placement information from the Stanford Research International survey, however, because of the likely variation of such placements across states.

Table 5-7.   Single federal handicap cost estimates per pupil ($),
California, 1988-1989

Federal handicap category	Age group	
	Five to seventeen (a)	Three to four (a)
Mentally retarded	11,499	13,021
Hard of hearing	12,896	13,887
Deaf	17,343	18,851
Speech impaired	2,550	2,642
Visually handicapped	21,944	22,953
Emotionally disturbed	14,177	16,051
Orthopedically handicapped	10,017	11,110
Other handicap	13,705	14,075
Learning disabled	4,317	4,843
Deaf and blind	17,914	19,487
Multiply handicapped	9,833	11,396

Note: Estimates based on regression results in Table 5-6 weighted by California special education enrollment by federal handicap and placement categories, 1988-1989 (see text).

(a) Costs for ages five to seventeen net out the displacement of regular education costs by placement category, as discussed in the text. Regular education costs for ages three to four are assumed to be zero.

(PCAFF) are given in Table 5-8 and range from $5,368 for those with cleft lip or palate[m] to $11,416 for those with Down syndrome.

Average special education utilization — Those with birth defects are not the exclusive recipients of special education. In order to make actual incremental cost estimates of the cost of special education, the probability of receiving special education among the general California population and its average cost should be

---

[m]Because there was insufficient data on the Stanford Research International survey to indicate the distribution of those with cleft lip or palate across federal handicap categories, we assumed that the distribution was the same as the California special education population as a whole. The incremental cost of special education for those with cleft lip or palate was, therefore, assigned the California average (see below).

Table 5-8.   Estimated special education cost per pupil ($) by
condition, 1988-1989

Condition	Age group	
	Five to seventeen (a)	Three to four (a)
Spina bifida	7,836	8,781
Conotruncal heart (a)	10,275	11,494
Cleft lip or palate	5,368	5,918
Limb reduction (b)	8,694	9,656
Down syndrome	11,416	12,940
Cerebral palsy	9,634	10,906
Average California	5,368	5,918

Note: Figures based on cost estimates of each handicap category (Table 5-7) weighted by the distribution across federal
handicap category by birth defect (Table 5-5). "Average California" is based upon distribution of all special education
students among federal handicap categories from the California Department of Education.

(a) Truncus arteriosus, transposition/DORV, tetralogy of Fallot, and single ventricle.

(b) Upper-limb reduction and lower-limb reduction.

considered. Based upon California special education enrollment as
a percentage of overall enrollment figures, there was a 9.5% chance
(p_i) that a student in California received special education in fiscal
year 1988-1989. Four-fifths of this special education population were
in two federal handicap categories: (a) learning disabled (56.1%) and
(b) speech impaired (25.9%). We determined an average cost of
special education (PCAFF) ($5,368) in the same manner as we
calculated the cost associated with each birth defect category by
multiplying the overall California enrollment proportions across
federal handicap categories by their respective costs from the
regressions reported above.   The higher than average per-pupil
special education cost estimates for every birth defect category,
except cleft deformity,[n] reflect the more costly federal handicap and
placement categories into which they fall.

Following Equation 5-1, we multiplied the proportion of those with
each birth defect (ages six to seventeen) receiving special education,

[n]See footnote m.

as reported above (p_i), by the size of the cohort alive at these ages (S_i) (Table 3-5) to arrive at a special education cohort by age for each birth defect category. This cohort estimate was multiplied by the per-capita cost estimate for each respective birth defect in Table 5-8 (PCAFF) to generate a total special education cost by age. We subtracted from this figure the average cost of special education ($5,368) for the 9.5% of the cohort at each age that would have been expected to have received special education.° These age-specific net costs were discounted to the first year of life and summed according to Equation 2-1, along with an estimate of special education for those ages 3-5 to arrive at an estimate of the total cost of special education by birth defect category.

Costs of Special Education Among Those Ages Three to Five

In recent years, there has been a large expansion of preschool programs for handicapped children. In order to continue to qualify for federal financing of special education, states had to enact laws by July 1, 1991, that entitled every developmentally delayed or disabled child from three through five years old to a range of preschool programs.[17] As of that date, all of the states but Oregon and Alabama provided extensive free preschool education for individuals. A lower percentage of handicapped preschool children, however, received special education than those of regular school age. We would have overestimated the proportion of those ages three to five within birth defect categories of interest who receive special education if we had routinely applied the overall proportion from the NHIS. We, therefore, made an estimate for three through five year-olds separately, based upon an analysis of enrollment by relevant federal handicap categories.

An estimate was made of those placed in each federal handicap category between the ages of six and ten in California as a percentage of the total school population between those ages. Similar

---

°We assumed that at least 9.5% of those in each birth defect cohort received special education, which is the rate in the general California population. For heart defects in which the estimated proportion receiving special education from the NHIS (7.7%) was below 9.5%, we assumed that the difference (1.8%) received special education at the average cost for California rather than the higher estimated cost for those with congenital heart defects.

percentages within the federal handicap category were made for three, four, and five year-olds separately. The latter percentages were divided by the former to determine the rate by which those in the federal handicap category receive preschool education at three, four, and five years old. For those in the mental retardation category, for example, the estimated rates at three, four and five years old were fairly high (62%, 83%, and 88%, respectively) of the percentage of mentally retarded students six to ten receiving special education. For children in learning disabled placement, however, preschool is even more rare; 7%, 13%, and 14% were the corresponding rates.

An underlying assumption of our method was that disabilities for which students received special education at ages six to ten were diagnosed by age three; thus, it was strictly the severity of the condition that served as the basis of deciding in favor or against early special education. To the extent that children are initially diagnosed after age three with learning disabilities, our method likely underestimates the percentage of those with birth defects who receive preschool special education by federal handicap category because those born with the structural congenital anomalies that drew our focus are likely diagnosed relatively early.

Preschool rates weighted by the estimated distribution among federal handicap categories (fc_j) in Table 5-5 were estimated for each birth defect category at age three, four, and five.[P] These percentages were multiplied by the estimated proportion receiving special education for each birth defect category (p) in order to estimate the size of the cohort at each preschool age receiving special education. The preschool rates for Down syndrome (for example, weighted heavily by the rates for the mental retardation federal handicap category) were 64%, 84%, and 89% for ages three, four, and five, respectively. Thus, rather than the proportion of five year-olds with Down syndrome requiring special education (p) at 83%, it was estimated at 74% (.89 x .83).

Even though five year-olds generally receive regular education, three and four year-olds generally do not. Consequently, we eliminated the "displacement cost" factor for regular education for three and four year-olds integrated into the cost estimates for five to

---

[P]Once again, the overall average for California was used for cleft lip or palate.

seventeen year-olds above. However, we reestimated the percentage of those receiving special education among the general school population (ages three, four, and five separately) and subtracted this percentage multiplied by the average estimated cost of special preschool education, as above, to generate the incremental cost of preschool special education for those with birth defects.[q,18,19]

Results

The total costs of special education by birth defect category are provided in Table 5-9. Total costs are highest for Down syndrome and cerebral palsy ($37.1 million and $28.6 million, respectively) at a 5% discount rate. These estimated costs of special education are approximately 85% higher than total net inpatient and outpatient medical care costs in the case of Down syndrome and about the same as those costs for those with cerebral palsy. The considerable total special education costs for these two conditions reflect a combination of three factors: (a) the relatively large incidence and survival to school age of those born with these conditions, (b) the high estimated proportions of those with each condition receiving special education (p_i), and (c) the high estimated average per-capita expense of the handicap and placement categories ($PCFC_{jk}$) into which those with these conditions fall. The relatively low total special education costs related to heart defects, in contrast, reflect (a) the far lower incidence of these conditions (and lower probability of survival to school age) and (b) the much smaller estimated proportion of those with congenital heart anomalies receiving special education (p_i).

Per-capita costs in the final column of Table 5-9 are total costs divided by the cohort at birth for each birth defect category. The patterns for per-capita costs are similar to those for total costs, with the exception that cleft lip or palate has a relatively low per-capita cost compared to total cost. Total cost reflects the large incidence of

---

[q]The base for preschool special education cost estimates was the same as for K-12 based on studies indicating that special preschool education can be more costly than K-12 special education. The *New York Times* reported a range of *average* preschool special education costs from $5,800 in a "typical" state such as Iowa to $14,700 in New York. Our cost estimates for three and four year-olds in California with birth defects range from $5,918 for those with cleft lip or palate to $12,940 for those with Down syndrome.

Table 5-9. Total and per-capita costs of special education services by condition in California, 1988-1989 (FY)

Condition	Total cost by discount rate ($000s)			Cost per case (a) by discount rate ($)		
	2%	5%	10%	2%	5%	10%
Spina bifida	6,972	5,264	3,458	30,805	23,261	15,278
Truncus arteriosus	99	76	51	1,772	1,353	906
Transposition/DORV	729	556	371	2,771	2,113	1,411
Tetralogy of Fallot	659	502	336	3,523	2,686	1,794
Single ventricle	145	110	74	2,130	1,624	1,085
Cleft lip or palate	2,992	2,217	1,407	3,169	2,348	1,490
Upper-limb reduction	4,033	3,067	2,039	17,232	13,103	8,711
Lower-limb reduction	1,969	1,497	995	17,208	13,081	8,692
Down syndrome	48,824	37,133	24,678	87,544	66,580	44,249
Cerebral palsy	37,691	28,639	19,008	57,368	43,591	28,931

Note: Figures are provided only for conditions for which there was an expectation of above-average rates of disability (those listed in quadrants II and IV of Table 2-2). Data limitations prevented us from estimating special education services' costs associated with renal agenesis.

(a) Cost-per-case estimated are total cost estimates divided by the number of individuals born with each condition in 1988 in California.

cleft lip or palate, whereas per-capita cost reflects a relatively low proportion receiving special education (p_i) coupled with a relatively low estimated per-pupil special education cost (PCAFF) among those with this congenital anomaly.

Endnotes to Chapter 5

1.California Department of Developmental Services. *Californians with Developmental Disabilities*; p. 22.

2.US Department of Education. *To Assure the Free Appropriate Public Education of All Children With Disabilities*. Thirteenth Annual Report to Congress of the Implementation of the Individuals with Disabilities Education Act.

3.Ibid.

4.Raphael ES, Singer JD, Walker DK. Per pupil expenditures on special education in three metropolitan school districts. *J Educ Fin*. 1985;1(Summer):69-88.

5.Lewis DR, Bruininks RH, Thurlow ML. Cost analysis of special schools for students with mental retardation. *J Spec Educ*. 1990;24(1):33-49.

6.Raphael ES, et al. Ibid.

7.Kakalik JS, Furry WS, Thomas MA, Carney MF. *The Cost of Special Education*. Santa Monica, California: Rand; 1981.

8.Moore MT, Strang EW, Schwartz M, Braddock M. *Patterns in Special Education Service Delivery and Cost*. Washington, DC: Decision Resources Corporation; 1988.

9.Kakalik JS, et al. Ibid.

10.Moore MT, et al. Ibid.

11.Kakalik JS, et al. Ibid.

12.Moore MT, et al. Ibid.

13.Chaikind S, Corman H. The impact of low birthweight on special education costs. *J Helth Econ*. 1991;10:291-311.

14.Ibid.

15.US Department of Education. Ibid.

16.Moore MT, et al. Ibid.

17.Nationwide revolution in education is giving handicapped a head start. *New York Times*; July 17, 1991:B7.

18.Moore MT, et al. Ibid.:107.

19.Nationwide revolution. Ibid.

Chapter 6

The Indirect Costs of Birth Defects: Premature Mortality and Heightened Morbidity

Introduction

In Chapters 4 and 5, we provided estimates of the societal costs associated with medical, educational, and developmental resources used by individuals born with at least one of eighteen birth defects. In the cost-of-illness literature, resources *used* are categorized as direct costs. Additional costs are associated with productivity *lost* to society due to premature mortality and heightened morbidity. A child born with spina bifida, for example, has a higher probability of early death or suffering from a work disability in adulthood than does the average child. The consequent loss to society of goods and services over the life course has a value that can be estimated. These lost resources are described in the cost-of-illness literature as indirect costs.[a]

---

[a] It should be emphasized that we are not estimating the value to society of the person, an exercise that is fraught with philosophical and ethical implications. Instead, we make an estimate of the lost economic product only. See Chapter 2 for a fuller discussion of cost-of-illness methodology and the calculation of indirect cost.

In this chapter, we describe our application of available data to the general method outlined in Chapter 2 and the resultant estimates of indirect costs of the birth defects of interest. After a discussion of the nature of indirect costs and the economic data used for their estimation, the remainder of the chapter is divided into two sections: (a) the indirect costs associated with premature mortality and (b) the indirect costs associated with premature morbidity.

Indirect Cost Methodology and Data

Under economic theory, earnings are viewed as returns to investments in training and education and other forms of "human capital." The estimation of lost earnings in cost-of-illness studies, as undertaken below, has, therefore, come to be known as the "human capital" approach. It is an estimate of the societal loss of economic product due to premature death and heightened morbidity.

In addition to lost earnings, economists also have undertaken the valuation of lost household production resulting from illness. For a premature death at age thirty-five, for example, the lost product to society is the earnings and household production that would have been produced from age thirty-five onward had the person lived an average life span.

General Method

We use the standard methodology of utilizing a cross-sectional profile of earnings and household production by age and sex to estimate the age-sex profile of earnings over the life course. This method assumes that the earnings and labor force participation rates by sex of infants today will be similar at each age in the future to their corresponding age and sex counterparts today. To the extent that females or males today will have higher sex-specific labor force participation rates and earnings forty years from now, for example, than their forty-year-old counterparts today, we underestimated the value of lifetime earnings for this particular age-sex group.

As has become customary in cost-of-illness studies, one adjustment to the cross-sectional age-sex-earnings profile that is reflected in our estimates is the integration of a 1% annual increase in labor productivity. Sixty-two year-olds in the year 2050, in other words, were projected to receive earnings that reflect a 1% annual compounded increase in real productivity since 1988 relative to sixty-two year-olds in 1988. If the actual average real annual productivity growth is under the projected 1% rate during the period from 1988 to 2050, then our estimates of indirect costs will be too high. On the other hand, if actual productivity turns out to be higher, then our estimates will be too low.

The incidence approach undertaken for this study required that we estimate indirect costs for the incident cases in the base year 1988. Because all incident cases of birth anomalies were less than age one by definition in the base year, the stream of indirect costs that we estimated began as of the year 2003 when the cohort started to enter the labor force in significant numbers at age fifteen and continued through 2053 when the cohort reached age sixty-five. Given the above annual 1% productivity adjustment, these age-specific earnings were higher than corresponding age-specific earnings in the base year. However, as in the case with direct costs, all future indirect costs (lost earnings and household production) were discounted back to the base year to estimate present value. Because we estimated costs associated with a birth cohort, all costs were discounted back to birth. The net effect of these two adjustments, discounting and productivity growth, is roughly the difference between the two. With our discount rate of 5%, for example, the net adjustment with a 1% productivity growth assumption is a 4% net discount.

To illustrate the net differences brought about by assumptions regarding productivity growth and discounting, the annual mean earnings of a sixty-two-year-old male in California in 1989 was $50,097 based upon US Bureau of the Census data. With a 1% annual increase in productivity, a male born in 1989 would earn $91,693 at age sixty-two in the year 2050, more than 80% higher than his counterpart in 1989. When discounted at 4% back to age zero, however, earnings at age sixty-two translate into a present value of only $17,569. Because the bulk of one's earnings is distant from birth, indirect costs of birth defects under an incidence approach are discounted heavily and, therefore, tend to be smaller than under a prevalence approach in which costs are calculated for all prevalent cases, spanning all ages, in a specific year.[b]

Earnings and Household Production Data

The age-sex profile of labor market earnings and value of household production used for the current study were drawn from detailed tables generated by Rice and Max for their study of the cost of smoking in California.[1] Annual mean compensation by age and gender in these tables were based on data from the US Bureau of the Census. The figures incorporated a broad package of compensation, including employer-provided supplements such as contributions for social security, health insurance, and private pensions in addition to wages and salary. In order to derive California-specific estimates, Rice and Max made a single adjustment to these national figures based on aggregate earnings data for California relative to the United States as a whole.

The California-detailed, age-sex profile of earnings for those less than one year-old in 1988, which forms the basis for all indirect cost calculations in this chapter, is provided by sex in Table 6-1. These figures are the 1989 figures from Rice and Max adjusted to 1988 compensation levels based on nominal changes in compensation in the United States between 1988 and 1989 from the US Bureau of Labor Statistics.[2]

Annual mean earnings through age sixty-five are provided in the third column of Table 6-1.[c] These earning figures incorporate the assumption of a 1% annual growth in productivity, as discussed above. Each figure can be looked upon as earnings in a future year in which the year is calculated as 1988 plus the age in column 1.

---

[b]See Chapter 2 for a discussion of the two approaches and the underlying rationale for choosing the incidence approach in this study.

[c]Rice and Max provide estimates through age ninety-nine, whereas we estimate indirect costs through age sixty-five. Because we discount all costs back to birth, the already reduced aggregate earnings in the table after age sixty-five because of higher rates of mortality and lower rates of labor-force participation are further diminished. The additional losses past usual retirement age, therefore, tend to be trivial. We estimate the mean earnings at age sixty-five using a linear smoothing function on earnings for the five-year age groups at approximately age sixty-five.

If we were to multiply the mean earnings in column 3 of Table 6-1 by the number of years in each age group in column 1 (five years in most cases), we would overestimate average aggregate earnings for the age group in the population because only a proportion of the general population survives to each age; among survivors, labor force participation is less than 100%. Adjustments for average survival and labor force participation patterns by sex and age are incorporated into the second column of Table 6-1, "Years of Earnings." Years of earnings by age substantially increase after the teen years, reflecting the fact that labor market participation begins to displace full-time school attendance as the norm. Declining values beyond ages forty to forty-four reflect decreasing life expectancy and increasing rates of retirement. Life expectancy data that are incorporated into column 2 of Table 6-1 are California-specific rates from the California Department of Health Services.[3] Labor-force participation rates incorporated into column 2 are percentages of the United States population by age and sex, with earnings in 1989 from the US Department of Labor.[4] Labor-force participation rates for California are assumed to be the same as those for the nation as a whole.

Average aggregate earnings per person by age group in column 4 of Table 6-1 is the product of columns 2 and 3. The lower aggregate earnings of females than of males reflect lower average mean earnings and lower average rates of labor-force participation in those age groups among females than among males. The final three columns of Table 6-1 reflect the aggregate earnings by age in column 4 discounted by 2%, 5%, and 10%, respectively, back to birth. The summation of the age entries in these columns by sex yield total present discounted value of expected future earnings.

The valuation of household production by age and sex are similarly adopted from Rice and Max.[5] They are based on time and motion studies of the household tasks performed and the market wages paid for these services, as developed by Douglass, Kenny, and Miller.[6]

The household production counterparts by sex to the detailed earnings' profile in Table 6-1 are not shown. Table 6-2 presents the final totals by age and sex of earnings and household production. Household production equals these totals minus the corresponding earning estimates in columns 5-7 of Table 6-1. All estimates of indirect costs due to birth defects in the remainder of the chapter utilize these figures or adjustments to these figures (discussed below).

The Cost of Birth Defects

Table 6-1. Estimates of average years of earnings, annual earnings, and present value of average lifetime earnings by age, sex, and discount rate for a person under age one in California, 1988

Age in years	Years of earnings	Annual mean earnings ($)	Aggregate earnings ($)	Present value of earnings ($) discounted at 2%	5%	10%
Males						
Less than 15	0.00	0	0	0	0	0
15-19	2.32	19,379	45,041	32,167	19,651	8,911
20-24	4.19	29,636	124,206	80,341	42,460	15,258
25-29	4.56	40,697	185,417	108,629	49,664	14,143
30-34	4.57	50,805	231,966	123,089	48,682	10,986
35-39	4.48	64,465	288,859	138,829	47,499	8,495
40-44	4.39	74,339	326,301	142,040	42,041	5,958
45-49	4.23	81,728	345,613	136,264	34,889	3,919
50-54	3.96	83,513	330,712	118,098	26,158	2,328
55-59	3.38	83,240	281,075	90,910	17,419	1,229
60-64	2.18	88,936	193,889	56,799	9,415	526
65	0.29	93,617	26,774	7,391	1,123	55
Total	N/A	N/A	2,379,854	1,034,557	339,001	71,809

Table 6-1.   (Continued)

Age in years	Years of earnings	Annual mean earnings ($)	Aggregate earnings ($)	Present value of earnings ($) discounted at		
				2%	5%	10%
Females						
Less than 15	0.00	0	0	0	0	0
15-19	2.19	18,029	39,440	28,167	17,208	7,803
20-24	3.59	25,070	90,008	58,221	30,769	11,057
25-29	3.65	32,094	117,262	68,699	31,408	8,944
30-34	3.60	37,758	135,968	72,149	28,535	6,440
35-39	3.68	41,334	152,017	73,061	24,997	4,471
40-44	3.76	44,607	167,808	73,047	21,620	3,064
45-49	3.58	46,038	165,004	65,056	16,657	1,871
50-54	3.13	44,868	140,289	50,097	11,096	988
55-59	2.54	45,096	114,350	36,985	7,087	500
60-64	1.58	47,201	74,587	21,850	3,622	202
65	0.21	49,497	10,355	2,858	434	21
Total	N/A	N/A	1,207,088	550,192	193,434	45,361

Note: Figures are based on the age-sex profile of labor force participation and earnings in 1988. Figures in the last three columns represent projected future earnings through age sixty-five of individuals born in 1988 in California discounted back to the year of birth, 1988. An annual real increase in productivity of 1% is assumed and incorporated in the table.

Indirect Costs of Birth Defects Due to Premature Mortality

We estimated lost earnings due to premature deaths based on Equation 2-2 reprinted here with slight modification as Equation 6-1:

$$TC_{ij} = (I-S_i) \times (PCPREV_{ij}), \qquad [6-1]$$

where $I-S_i$ is an estimate of those who prematurely die in the birth cohort by age i, and the per-capita cost of such mortality at age i

Table 6-2. Estimated average discounted future earnings and imputed value of household production ($) for a person under age one in California in 1988 by age, sex, and discount rate

Age in years	Earnings discounted at		
	2%	5%	10%
Males			
Less than 15	0	0	0
15-19	36,554	22,332	10,127
20-24	91,675	48,449	17,411
25-29	122,188	55,863	15,909
30-34	137,519	54,389	12,274
35-39	153,197	52,415	9,374
40-44	155,804	46,114	6,536
45-49	148,962	38,141	4,284
50-54	129,452	28,673	2,552
55-59	100,383	19,234	1,357
60-64	62,719	10,396	581
65	8,174	1,242	60
Total	1,146,628	377,248	80,464

Table 6-2. (Continued)

Age in years	Earnings discounted at		
	2%	5%	10%
Females			
Less than 15	0	0	0
15-19	40,466	24,722	11,210
20-24	83,634	44,200	15,884
25-29	102,943	47,064	13,403
30-34	109,907	43,469	9,810
35-39	109,627	37,508	6,708
40-44	106,261	31,451	4,457
45-49	94,596	24,221	2,720
50-54	78,426	17,371	1,546
55-59	63,299	12,129	856
60-64	45,015	7,462	417
65	6,997	1,063	52
Total	841,172	290,658	67,063

($PCPREV_{ij}$) is average age- and sex-specific earnings of the general population.[d] Two sets of information are, therefore, required for such estimates: (a) the survival profile of those with conditions of interest to estimate $I-S_i$ and (b) the labor force and earnings' profile of the general population by age and sex to estimate $PCPREV_{ij}$. The latter set of information has been discussed and presented above (Table 6-2). The estimated value of lost household and market production ($PCPREV_{ij}$) from the death of a male infant ($i=0$) discounted at 5%, for example, is the sum of all figures in column 2 of Table 6-2 ($377,248). For someone dying at age twenty-four ($i=24$) in the year 2012, the analogous indirect cost to society is the

---

[d]The number of survivors, S_i, in Equation 6-2, in other words, is replaced in this instance by $I-S_i$, the number of deaths by age i.

sum of entries ages twenty-five to twenty-nine through age sixty-five ($306,567).

The mortality profile of those with birth defects is based on the survival estimates by condition, for which selected entries were provided in Table 3-5. For each condition, normal survival was assumed after a particular age, as described in Chapter 2. We calculated indirect costs due to mortality by condition only for deaths up to the age at which the normal survival curve was introduced, that is, only for the period in which we had information on excess mortality. For all birth conditions except those listed in quadrant IV of Table 2-2, this period is the first year of life only. As discussed in Chapter 3, data limitations also prevented us from constructing the mortality profile past infancy for conotruncal heart anomalies and for renal agenesis or dysgenesis. For those born with spina bifida, cerebral palsy, or Down syndrome, the age cutoffs for excess mortality are nine years, seventeen years, and sixty-five years, respectively.[e]

A detailed profile of indirect mortality costs for spina bifida is provided in Table 6-3 as an example of our methodology. The first three columns of the table provide cohort estimates, age-specific deaths, and cumulative deaths by age group. The cohort estimates in the table are the number alive at birth for the zero to fourteen age group and the number alive at the midpoint of each five-year age group until age sixty-five in which the entry is the estimated number alive at sixty-five. More specifically, the cohort estimate for spina bifida in the age fifteen to nineteen group is the number born in 1988 with the condition who are estimated to be alive at age seventeen and so on. Age-specific death entries in the second column are the numbers who die through the year prior to reaching the age of the next cohort estimate. Deaths from age zero to fourteen are indicated next to the "under fifteen age category," deaths from age fifteen to sixteen are entered in the fifteen to nineteen category, deaths from seventeen to twenty-one in the twenty to twenty-four category, and so on. Because excess deaths for all conditions except cerebral palsy and Down syndrome were estimated to be prior to age seventeen, there are no nonzero entries in this column after the under fifteen

---

[e]For Down syndrome, we have information on mortality through age sixty-seven but, as noted earlier, we calculate indirect costs only through age sixty-five.

category for any of the other conditions, including spina bifida.

Age-specific deaths were added successively to arrive at cumulative deaths in column 3 of Table 6-3. For the same reason that there are no nonzero entries after the first row, entries in the third column are constant at the number of excess deaths prior to age fifteen for all conditions, except cerebral palsy and Down syndrome as well. Deaths through age sixteen were recorded in the cumulative death column next to the age fifteen to nineteen entry, through age twenty-one next to the twenty to twenty-four entry, through twenty-six opposite the twenty-five to twenty-nine entry, and so on. The use of the midpoint of each age group as a cutoff resulted in slight underestimates of indirect mortality costs for cerebral palsy and larger underestimates for Down syndrome. This was due to the assignment of those dying in the latter three years of each of five-year grouping to the subsequent five-year group. By doing so, however, we remained consistent in our estimation of the size of the cohort alive in each age group and, thereby, avoided double-counting in our calculations of indirect costs due to morbidity.

The product of the age-specific cumulative death total and the discounted aggregate earnings yielded the total economic loss attributable to mortality from spina bifida by age group (columns 4-6 of Table 6-3). The sum of these entries yielded the total indirect mortality costs for spina bifida for each discount rate (last row).

The corresponding summary indirect mortality cost totals for each condition by discount rate is provided in Table 6-4.

Indirect Costs of Birth Defects Due to Heightened Morbidity

People with birth defects may have disabilities arising directly from their birth anomalies or from associated conditions that create limitations in their ability to work. These disabilities may render them (a) totally unable to work or (b) limited in the amount or type of work they can perform. These two levels of limitation lent themselves to separate treatment in our analysis. We made estimates of the costs for each morbidity component, however, based on general Equation 2-4 and reprinted here as Equation 6-2:

Table 6-3. Indirect mortality costs and years of lost earnings due to mortality for the cohort born with spina bifida in California in 1988 by age, sex, and discount rate

Age in years	Size of cohort (S,)	Excess mortality	Cumulative excess mortality	Present value of indirect mortality costs ($1,000s) discounted at			Years of lost earnings
				2%	5%	10%	
Males							
Less than 15	108	27	27	0	0	0	0
15-19	81	0	27	987	603	273	63
20-24	80	0	27	2,475	1,308	470	113
25-29	80	0	27	3,299	1,508	430	123
30-34	79	0	27	3,713	1,469	331	123
35-39	78	0	27	4,136	1,415	253	121
40-44	77	0	27	4,207	1,245	176	119
45-49	75	0	27	4,023	1,030	116	114
50-54	73	0	27	3,495	774	69	107
55-59	70	0	27	2,710	519	37	91
60-64	65	0	27	1,693	281	16	59
65	61	0	27	221	34	2	25
Total	N/A	27	N/A	30,960	10,186	2,173	1,058

Table 6-3. (Continued)

Age in years	Size of cohort (S_i)	Excess mortality	Cumulative excess mortality	Present value of indirect mortality costs ($1,000s) discounted at			Years of lost earnings
				2%	5%	10%	
Females							
Less than 15	119	29	29	0	0	0	0
15-19	90	0	29	1,174	717	325	63
20-24	89	0	29	2,425	1,282	461	104
25-29	89	0	29	2,985	1,365	389	106
30-34	89	0	29	3,187	1,261	284	104
35-39	88	0	29	3,179	1,088	195	107
40-44	88	0	29	3,082	912	129	109
45-49	87	0	29	2,743	702	79	104
50-54	85	0	29	2,274	504	45	91
55-59	83	0	29	1,836	352	25	74
60-64	80	0	29	1,305	216	12	46
65	77	0	29	203	31	2	6
Total	N/A	29	N/A	24,394	8,429	1,945	914
Grand total (males plus female)							
0 65	N/A	56	N/A	55,353	18,615	4,117	1,972

Note: While there may be excess mortality/below-normal survival after age nine for individuals with spina bifida, there has been little recent reliable data on such mortality in the clinical literature. Column sums may not equal column totals due to rounding.

Table 6-4. Summary indirect mortality costs of birth defects in California by condition, sex, and discount rate ($1,000s, 1988)

Condition	2% discount			5% discount			10% discount		
	Male	Female	Total	Male	Female	Total	Male	Female	Total
Spina bifida	30,959	24,394	55,352	10,186	8,429	18,615	2,173	1,944	4,117
Truncus arteriosus	22,933	12,618	35,550	7,545	4,360	11,905	1,609	1,006	2,615
Transposition/DORV	76,824	32,806	109,630	25,276	11,336	36,611	5,391	2,616	8,007
Tetralogy of Fallot	29,812	16,823	46,636	9,809	5,813	15,622	2,092	1,341	3,433
Single ventricle	24,079	13,459	37,538	7,922	4,651	12,573	1,690	1,073	2,763
Cleft lip or palate	83,704	50,470	134,174	27,539	17,440	44,979	5,874	4,024	9,898
TE fistula	22,933	15,982	38,915	7,545	5,523	13,068	1,609	1,274	2,883
Atresia, small intestine	9,173	8,411	17,585	3,018	2,907	5,925	644	671	1,314
Colorectal atresia	40,132	21,029	61,161	13,204	7,266	20,470	2,816	1,677	4,493
Renal agenesis	110,076	41,217	151,294	36,216	14,242	50,458	7,725	3,286	11,011
Urinary obstruction	84,851	27,759	112,609	27,916	9,592	37,508	5,954	2,213	8,167
Upper-limb reduction	20,639	13,459	34,098	6,791	4,651	11,441	1,448	1,073	2,521
Lower-limb reduction	14,906	7,571	22,477	4,904	2,616	7,520	1,046	604	1,650
Diaphragmatic hernia	73,384	40,376	113,760	24,144	13,952	38,095	5,150	3,219	8,369

Table 6-4. (Continued)

Condition	2% discount			5% discount			10% discount		
	Male	Female	Total	Male	Female	Total	Male	Female	Total
Gastroschisis	13,760	6,729	20,489	4,527	2,325	6,852	966	537	1,502
Omphalocele	24,079	15,141	39,220	7,922	5,232	13,154	1,690	1,207	2,897
Down syndrome	103,153	73,102	176,254	30,749	22,776	53,525	5,838	4,690	10,527
Cerebral palsy	50,415	28,559	78,974	16,577	9,858	26,434	3,530	2,269	5,799

Note: Mortality costs reflect lifetime productivity loss due to excess first-year mortality for all birth defects except for three listed in quadrant IV of Table 2-2: spina bifida (through age nine), Down syndrome (through age sixty-five), and cerebral palsy (through age seventeen). While excess mortality beyond the first year is likely for other conditions listed in that quadrant, data limitations prevented us from making such estimates (see note to Table 2-2).

$$TC_{ij} = (S_i) \times (p_{ij}) \times (PCAFF_{ij}), \hspace{2cm} [6\text{-}2]$$

where p_{ij} is the proportion of the prevalent population with the defect that is unable to work (j=unable) or limited in the amount or type of work they can perform (j=limited in amount or type) at age i.

Costs Due To Total Disability

An estimate of those unable to work by condition (p_{ij}) was sufficient when coupled with the full earnings' profile above ($PCAFF_{ij}$) and estimates of survival in Chapter 3 (S_i) to generate estimates of indirect costs arising from this level of disability. Additional information was required to estimate costs due to partial work limitation, as discussed below. For both categories of estimates, we assumed that there are concomitant reductions in household production to labor market earnings due to these limitations.

The pooled sample from the 1985-1989 National Health Interview Surveys, used to make prevalence estimates for several of the conditions beyond age one (Chapter 3) and estimates of special education enrollment (Chapter 5), also was used to assess the extent of work limitations by condition for several of the birth defects (p_{ij}). All respondents ages eighteen to sixty-five on the National Health Interview Surveys are queried with respect to their work limitations, that is, whether they were unable to work or were limited in the amount or type of work they can perform.[f] We generated our estimates of the percentages of those unable to work by condition based on responses to this question.

An objection might be raised concerning limitations not directly related to the underlying condition of interest. Someone born with a cleft lip or palate, for example, may have a work limitation not directly related to their birth anomaly. As noted in Chapter 2, we attempted to estimate the incremental cost for people with conditions, not the incremental costs of conditions per se. To the extent those born with a cleft lip or palate have higher rates of work limitations than the average person, regardless of whether they are directly due to cleft lip or palate or to associated anomalies that may

---

[f]See Appendix 2 for a description of the National Health Interview Surveys pooled sample.

or may not be well-understood, such limitations were counted as indirect costs for people with these conditions. Consequently, we calculated the full proportion unable to work by condition and subtracted the overall rate of limitation in the population, as derived from the National Health Interview Surveys sample. The result was an estimate of the incremental rate of limitation among those with birth conditions of interest.

Estimates from the National Health Interview Surveys sample on rates of total and partial work disability among the noninstitutionalized United States population eighteen to sixty-five for those with conditions listed in quadrants II or IV of Table 2-2 are provided in Table 6-5. The fact that there were significant numbers with Down syndrome and cerebral palsy who resided in developmental centers and other long-term care facilities (see Chapter 4) suggests that our estimates of work limitations from the National Health Interview Surveys may be too low. Our indirect cost estimates for these conditions, in particular, may be downwardly biased.

As with estimates of special education requirements from this survey, we had to rely on aggregated National Health Interview Surveys categories to make estimates of p_{ij} for certain conditions. The level of work disability for Down syndrome was based upon the rates among those with congenital mental retardation, whereas the rates for each heart anomaly is based upon the average of a larger group of congenital heart defects than those we estimated (International Classification of Diseases, 9th Revision [ICD-9]:745-746). The aggregated categories are the respective "Recode C" categories on National Health Interview Surveys into which they are folded (Appendix 2). For chronic conditions such as cerebral palsy, Down syndrome, and spina bifida, rates of disability were understandably the highest.

The National Health Interview Surveys inquired as to whether one's work limitation is mainly, secondarily, or not attributable to the underlying condition. The percentages for which the underlying condition was reported as the primary or secondary cause of the work limitation are reported in parentheses in Table 6-5. The latter proportion was nearly the entire total for defects such as cerebral palsy, Down syndrome, spina bifida, and limb reductions. For cleft lip or palate and congenital heart defects, on the other hand, the defect was listed as the primary or secondary cause in well below

The Cost of Birth Defects

Table 6-5. Work limitation rates and earnings reductions because of limitations in the amount or type of work

	Percent unable to work	Percent limited in amount or type of work	Percent reduction in earnings	
			Male	Female
US population	05.4	4.5		
Spina bifida	27.1 (19.5)	4.3 (00.0)		
Congenital heart (a)	15.7 (06.2)	12.4 (05.5)		
Cleft lip or palate	11.7 (02.0)	17.2 (00.0)		
Upper-limb reduction	14.0 (14.0)	. .		
Lower-limb reduction	35.2 (25.9)	13.5 (13.5)		
Congenital mental retardation (b)	62.9 (56.0)	29.1 (24.3)		
Cerebral palsy	62.9 (53.1)	15.1 (15.1)		
Limited (c)			46.0	17.0
Limited, mentally retarded (d)			70.0	45.0

Note: Figures on the proportion unable to work or limited in the amount or type of work are from the pooled 1985-1989 National Health Interview Survey (NHIS), ages eighteen to sixty-five. Numbers in parentheses indicate the corresponding percent limited in which the condition was listed as the main or secondary cause of the work limitation on the NHIS. (See text for more detail.) Figures on the reduction in earnings because of limitations in the amount or type of work are from the Survey of Income and Program Participation (SIPP), 1987. The "limited" figures reflect earnings for those who were limited prior to working age and whose limitations were not due to an accident. The "limited, mentally retarded" entries reflect an additional stipulation that the limiting condition is mental retardation.

(a) Estimates from congenital heart problems were used for conotruncal heart defects (common truncus, transposition/DORV, tetralogy of Fallot, and single ventricle).

(b) Figures used for Down syndrome.

(c) Figures used for all conditions, except Down syndrome, to estimate earnings reductions because of limitations in the amount or type of work.

(d) Figures used for Down syndrome only.

50% of the cases. Yet, the overall proportion of people with these conditions unable to work was well above the population as a whole. This finding reinforces the notion that people born with these defects had or developed associated conditions responsible for higher than expected levels of work limitations.

The difference between the condition-specific estimate and the United States population estimate in Table 6-5 is the proportion that we applied to the cohort alive in each age group to arrive at an incremental "unable to work" cohort by age for each condition. An illustration of our methodology for spina bifida is provided in Table 6-6. Column 3 of the table provides this "unable to work" cohort by sex. This cohort number was multiplied by the age-specific, discounted average earnings figure (Table 6-2), as with the indirect mortality cost estimates, to arrive at age- and sex-specific totals by the three discount rates (Table 6-6, columns 4-6). Column sums yielded the sex-specific estimates of indirect costs due to being unable to work. The addition across gender yielded total costs by condition. These summary totals for spina bifida are provided in the bottom row of Table 6-6 and for all relevant conditions in columns 1-3 of Table 6-7.

We applied the average estimate of limitation by condition, ages eighteen to sixty-five, from the National Health Interview Surveys to the age- and sex-specific cohort numbers in the earnings tables. The relatively small number of respondents in the pooled five-year National Health Interview Surveys sample with spina bifida and limb reduction, in particular, prevented us from utilizing more refined sex- and age-specific rates of work limitations for all conditions. Estimates from more refined age- and sex-specific rates for conditions in which refinement was possible, however, were not substantially different from the reported aggregate estimates in Table 6-7.

Costs From Limitations in the Amount or Type of Work

The same method and data used for estimating those unable to work were employed for making estimates of the proportion limited in amount or type of work (Table 6-5, columns 3-4). Additional information was required, however, to estimate the percentage reduction in earnings associated with limitations, thus making an accurate estimate of $PCAFF_{ij}$ in this instance. These percentage reductions are applied to the aggregate earnings figures in Table 6-2 to estimate indirect costs due to partial work limitations.

We used the 1987 Survey of Income and Program Participation, Wave 2, to estimate the percentage reduction in earnings due to work limitations. The Survey of Income and Program Participation is an annual cohort survey conducted by the US Bureau of the Census on a nationally representative sample of households and persons in the

Table 6-6. Indirect morbidity costs due to being unable to work for the cohort born with spina bifida in California in 1988 by age, sex, and discount rate

Age in years	Size of cohort (S$_i$)	Number unable to work (p$_i$ x S$_i$)	Present value or indirect mortality costs ($1,000s) discounted at		
			2%	5%	10%
Males					
Less than 15	108	N/A	0	0	0
15-19	81	17.6	643	393	178
20-24	80	17.4	1,592	841	302
25-29	80	17.4	2,121	970	276
30-34	79	17.1	2,358	932	210
35-39	78	16.9	2,593	887	159
40-44	77	16.7	2,603	771	109
45-49	75	16.3	2,424	621	70
50-54	73	15.8	2,051	454	40
55-59	70	15.2	1,525	292	21
60-64	65	14.1	885	147	8
65	61	13.2	108	16	1
Total	N/A	N/A	18,902	6,324	1,375

Table 6-6. (Continued)

Age in years	Size of cohort (S_i)	Number unable to work ($p_i \times S_i$)	Present value of indirect mortality costs ($1,000s) discounted at		
			2%	5%	10%
Females					
Less than 15	119	N/A	0	0	0
15-19	90	19.5	790	483	219
20-24	89	19.3	1,615	854	307
25-29	89	19.3	1,988	909	259
30-34	89	19.3	2,123	840	189
35-39	88	19.1	2,093	716	128
40-44	88	19.1	2,029	601	85
45-49	87	18.9	1,786	457	51
50-54	85	18.5	1,447	320	29
55-59	83	18.0	1,140	219	15
60-64	80	17.4	782	130	7
65	77	16.7	117	18	1
Total	N/A	N/A	15,910	5,545	1,291
Grand total (male plus female)					
0-65	N/A	N/A	34,812	11,869	2,665

Note: Estimates of the number of individuals with spina bifida unable to work in the third column of the table is based on the percentage unable to work with spina bifida (27.1) minus the average in the US population (5.4) from Table 6-5 multiplied by the estimated size of the cohort at each age (column 1). Column sums may not equal totals due to rounding.

Table 6-7. Summary indirect morbidity costs of birth defects in California by condition, degree of limitation, and discount rate ($1,000s, 1988)

Condition	Unable to work			Limited in work			Total: Unable plus limited		
	Lifetime costs discounted at			Lifetime costs discounted at			Lifetime costs discounted at		
	2%	5%	10%	2%	5%	10%	2%	5%	10%
Spina bifida	34,812	11,869	2,665	0	0	0	34,812	11,869	2,665
Truncus arteriosus	2,127	722	161	578	195	43	2,705	916	203
Transposition/DORV	15,691	5,318	1,182	4,452	1,499	329	20,143	6,817	1,512
Tetralogy of Fallot	13,984	4,750	1,060	3,790	1,277	281	17,774	6,027	1,341
Single ventricle	3,091	1,050	234	843	284	63	3,933	1,334	297
Cleft lip or palate	48,777	16,579	3,704	34,307	11,568	2,549	83,083	28,147	6,253
Upper-limb reduction	16,368	5,565	1,244	0	0	0	16,368	5,565	1,244
Lower-limb reduction	26,608	9,034	2,014	2,854	962	212	29,461	9,996	2,226
Down syndrome	217,239	76,255	17,583	55,224	19,286	4,412	273,463	95,541	21,995
Cerebral palsy	321,374	109,182	24,372	20,898	7,044	1,551	342,273	116,226	25,923

Note: Morbidity costs were estimated only for conditions listed in quadrants II and IV of Table 2-2. Data limitations prevented us from estimating morbidity costs associated with renal agenesis. While above-normal rates of limitations in the amount and type of work that can be performed may prevail for individuals with spina bifida and upper-limb reduction, our pooled NHIS sample did not reveal such rates (Table 6-5). Row totals may not equal row sums because of rounding.

United States. The cohort is followed over approximately two and a half years and is reinterviewed at five-month intervals. Each interview that provides information on labor force participation, income, wealth, and public program participation in the intervening four months is called a "Wave." In several Waves, "topical modules" are devoted to questions regarding special topics. In Wave 2 of the 1987 survey conducted between June and September 1987, a topical module was devoted to work disability. Respondents age sixteen to sixty-seven were queried with respect to their work limitations and conditions underlying their limitations. We used responses to this module in addition to general population earnings data from the survey to make estimates of percentage reductions in earnings because of limitations in the amount or type of work performed to estimate $PCAFF_{ij}$.

Categories of conditions underlying work limitations were too broadly defined on the Survey of Income and Program Participation to make estimates with respect to any specific condition of interest. However, the Survey of Income and Program Participation inquired as to the timing of the limitation, that is, whether it began before the respondent reached working age and whether it was because of an accident. Those responding (a) affirmatively to being limited prior to working age and (b) negatively to the limitation because of an accident were selected as the sample to estimate reductions in earnings due to work limitations arising from birth defects. Because one of the conditions on the Survey of Income and Program Participation condition list was mental retardation, we made estimates for those with Down syndrome based on "a" and "b" above, with the additional stipulation of being (c) listed as mentally retarded.

For respondents on the Survey of Income and Program Participation, ages sixteen to sixty-five, who were limited in the amount or type of work they could perform and who met the other conditions above, we calculated the mean monthly earnings over the previous four months and compared it to the corresponding earnings of their nonlimited counterparts. The percentage reduction in earnings by sex is provided in columns 5-6 of Table 6-5.

Note that we did not make the stipulation that respondents had to have earnings or had to be in the labor force during the period. Had we made such a stipulation we would have made the implicit assumption that labor-force participation rates and unemployment rates among those with work limitations were the same as those without. Without a restriction, we allowed for differences. It is not surprising, therefore, to find that earnings reductions due to being limited in amount or type of work among females is lower than among males. Females who are not limited are more likely to be married, have children, and have lower rates of labor-force participation than those who are limited. Those who are limited will have lower earnings and more restricted activity days than their counterparts with earnings, but their higher labor-force participation rates make up, in part, for reductions.

The National Health Interview Survey rates of being limited in the amount or type of work that can be performed by condition (p_{ij}) were multiplied by the cohort estimates (S_i) by condition to arrive at an "amount or type" cohort by age and sex, as with the "unable" cohort in the example for spina bifida above. These cohort products were multiplied by $PCAFF_{ij}$, the product of the corresponding discounted aggregate earnings figures (Table 6-2) and the percentage reduction in earnings from the Survey of Income and Program Participation (Table 6-5), to arrive at indirect costs by age group due to limitations in the amount or type of work that can be performed. These figures were summed over all ages, as above, to arrive at total estimates of indirect morbidity costs due to partial work limitations. These summary estimates are provided, by discount rate, in columns 4-6 of Table 6-7.

Results

Total indirect mortality costs of birth defects in California by sex and discount rate are provided in Table 6-4. Costs range from $5.9 million for atresia of the small intestine to $53.5 million for Down syndrome at a 5% discount rate. The high total cost for Down syndrome largely reflects the fact that costs were computed for excess mortality through age sixty-five, whereas for most conditions costs were computed for mortality through the first year of life only (see above). The effect of discounting on indirect costs in our study is particularly large, given that earnings are concentrated in adulthood and all costs are discounted back to birth.

The mortality costs associated with Down syndrome were largest, but the impact of discounting such costs also was greater for this condition because the future earnings stream of an adult tends to be small when discounted back to birth. The indirect mortality costs for excess adult mortality in the case of Down syndrome, therefore, becomes less significant the higher the discount rate. As an illustration, consider the difference in mortality costs of Down syndrome and renal agenesis (the next costly condition in terms of mortality) at different discount rates. Excess mortality through age sixty-five is incorporated into the analysis for Down syndrome and through the first year of life for renal agenesis. At a 2% discount rate, the indirect mortality costs of Down syndrome were approximately $25 million higher than renal agenesis, whereas the difference becomes negative and approximately $.5 million at a 10% discount rate.

The higher costs for males reflect the higher incidence of most of the diseases among males, as well as the higher lifetime profile of earnings of males relative to females.

Summary indirect morbidity cost estimates in Table 6-7 reveal that the highest costs because of the inability to work were incurred by those with Down syndrome and cerebral palsy ($76.3 million and $109.2 million, respectively) discounted at 5%. These costs reflect the relatively high incidence of these conditions, high survival into adulthood, and high rates of incapacity to work (Table 6-5) among adults with these conditions. The indirect morbidity costs due to limitations in the amount or type of work are nearly three times as high for Down syndrome ($19.3 million) than for cerebral palsy ($7 million); however, even though the incidence of cerebral palsy is higher than that of Down syndrome and the estimated rate of limitation (Table 6-5) of the latter condition is less than twice that of the former. This result is due to the higher estimated reduction in earnings (70%) for Down syndrome relative to cerebral palsy (46%). If those with cerebral palsy with work limitations have lower earnings than the estimate for the general population with limitations, then our estimate for indirect morbidity costs due to limitations in the amount or type of work for cerebral palsy is too low.

Summary indirect costs due to mortality and morbidity by condition and discount rate for California in 1988 are given in Table 6-8. A summary comparison of these costs to direct costs is provided in Chapter 7.

The Cost of Birth Defects

Table 6-8. Summary indirect costs of birth defects in California by condition and discount rate ($1,000s, 1988)

Condition	Total direct cost by discount rate		
	2%	5%	10%
Spina bifida	90,164	30,484	6,782
Truncus arteriosus	38,255	12,821	2,819
Transposition/DORV	129,773	43,428	9,518
Tetralogy of Fallot	64,410	21,649	4,774
Single ventricle	41,471	13,907	3,060
Cleft lip or palate	217,257	73,125	16,150
TE fistula	38,915	13,068	2,884
Atresia, small intestine	17,585	5,925	1,314
Colorectal atresia	61,161	20,470	4,493
Renal agenesis	151,294	50,458	11,011
Urinary obstruction	112,609	37,508	8,167
Upper-limb reduction	50,466	17,006	3,765
Lower-limb reduction	51,938	17,516	3,876
Diaphragmatic hernia	113,760	38,096	8,369
Gastroschisis	20,489	6,852	1,502
Omphalocele	39,220	13,154	2,897
Down syndrome	448,717	149,065	32,522
Cerebral palsy	421,247	142,661	31,723

Note: Indirect costs are mortality plus morbidity costs (Tables 6-4 and 6-7).

Endnotes to Chapter 6

1.Rice DP, Max W. *The Cost of Smoking in California, 1989.* Sacramento, California: California State Department of Health Services; 1992.

2.US Bureau of Labor Statistics. *Statistical Abstract of the United States.* Washington, DC: Author; 1991:Table 671.

3.California Department of Health Services. *Life Tables for California.* Sacramento, California: Author; 1991.

4.US Department of Labor, Bureau of Labor Statistics. *Employment and Earnings.* Washington, DC: Author; January 1990:162.

5.Rice DP, Max W. Ibid.

6.Douglass JB, Kenny GM, Miller TR. Which estimates of household production are best? *J Forensic Econ.* 1990;4(1):25-45.

Chapter 7

An Assessment of Total Costs and Policy Implications

Summary Costs

Our estimates of direct and indirect costs of birth defects in California, at a discount rate of 5%, ranged from $12.8 million for atresia of the small intestine to $292.1 million for cerebral palsy in 1988 (Table 7-1). These cost estimates by birth defect were particularly sensitive to the incidence of the defect in the population, the extent of premature mortality associated with the condition, and the degree to which the defect and/or associated anomalies were responsible for functional and activity limitations. The most costly conditions (cerebral palsy and Down syndrome) have relatively high incidence rates and very high rates of activity limitations among survivors. The high cost of cleft lip/palate reflects its high incidence rate, coupled with relatively high rates of first-year mortality and activity limitations into adulthood.

The summary total and per capita costs reported in Table 7-1 are indicative of large costs, whereas the breakdown of total cost into its various direct and indirect components (Table 7-2) reveals a diversity in disease patterns and associated treatment and cost profiles that could not be gleaned from an aggregate estimate such as that of Rice, Hodgson, and Kopstein.[1] High rates of activity limitations for chronic diseases such as cerebral palsy, Down syndrome, and spina

Table 7-1. Summary total costs and costs per case of birth defects in California by condition and discount rate ($1,000s, 1988)

Condition	Total cost by discount rate			Cost per case by discount rate		
	2%	5%	10%	2%	5%	10%
Spina bifida	126,357	58,375	27,406	558	258	121
Truncus arteriosus	51,209	24,681	13,678	907	437	242
Transposition/DORV	149,729	62,204	26,862	569	237	102
Tetralogy of Fallot	87,032	42,430	23,412	466	227	125
Single ventricle	51,026	20,772	8,264	747	304	121
Cleft lip or palate	232,183	86,352	27,493	246	91	29
TE fistula	45,741	19,811	9,499	295	128	61
Atresia, small intestine	24,598	12,843	8,087	123	64	40
Colorectal atresia	67,580	26,737	10,536	279	110	44
Renal agenesis	154,042	53,165	13,660	667	230	59
Urinary obstruction	117,745	42,579	13,138	212	77	24
Upper-limb reduction	55,735	21,292	6,999	238	91	30
Lower-limb reduction	56,690	20,826	6,174	495	182	54
Diaphragmatic hernia	120,696	44,971	15,153	610	227	77
Gastroschisis	26,540	12,824	7,353	195	94	54
Omphalocele	42,309	16,207	5,894	415	159	58
Down syndrome	568,690	228,731	85,142	1,020	410	153
Cerebral palsy	700,913	292,130	109,899	1,067	445	167

Note: Total costs represent the sum of direct and indirect lifetime costs associated with the cohort born in California in 1988. Figures represent costs discounted back to the year of birth (1988). Cost per case are total costs divided by the number of incident cases of each condition in 1988.

bifida translated into high nonmedical direct costs for special education and developmental services, as might be expected. Similarly, the ratio of long-term care costs to inpatient and outpatient medical costs for these defects was much larger than for other congenital anomalies in our study. Activity limitations also were responsible for the high estimated indirect costs related to morbidity for these conditions. This diversity among defects should help to inform policy in weighing prevention strategies, as discussed further below.

Projection of Costs to the United States

The costs of birth defects estimated in California projected to the nation are provided in Table 7-3. In order to make national cost projections from our California estimates, we adjusted for the estimated differences in the number of incident cases in California relative to the nation and also for cost differences between the two areas. We multiplied the aggregate estimates reported in Table 7-1 by the number of annual births in the United States relative to California in order to make a national estimate. We thereby assumed that the incidence of the birth defects we analyzed in the United States was similar to that of California.

We deflated this aggregate cost figure by the extent to which average employee compensation in California exceeded the national average in 1988 (1.103) based on the Statistical Abstract of the United States (1991).* The resulting national estimate of cost by birth defect, at a 5% discount rate, are provided in the first column of Table 7-3. An underlying assumption to this adjustment is that patterns of treatment in the nation for birth defects are similar to that in California.

In order to express these estimates in 1992 dollars, we inflated the estimated medical care component of these cost estimates by the increase in the medical care component of the consumer price

---

*This deflation factor is appropriate for indirect costs, which are computed from average compensation data in California. We believe that the use of this factor to deflate direct costs also was appropriate for several reasons. Direct education and developmental services costs are labor intensive and are largely provided through negotiated public contract. Inpatient medical care charges have been deflated considerably based upon Medicare's ratio of charge to cost index (Chapter 4). Physician costs were based on Medicare rates as well, whereas other medical direct costs were based on Medicaid-negotiated reimbursement (Chapter 4). The remaining difference in medical expenditures in California relative to the nation is likely to be related to differences in the cost of living. The deflation of direct medical cost estimates in California based on differences in average compensation, therefore, seemed appropriate.

Table 7-2. Summary cost of birth defects in California, by cost category, discounted at 5% ($1,000s, 1988)

Condition	Direct costs			Indirect costs		Total costs
	Medical (a)	Special education (b)	Developmental services (b)	Morbidity (c)	Mortality (c)	
Spina bifida	22,402	5,264	225	11,869	18,615	58,375
Truncus arteriosus	11,784	76	--	916	11,905	24,681
Transposition/DORV	18,220	556	--	6,817	36,611	62,204
Tetralogy of Fallot	20,279	502	--	6,027	15,622	42,430
Single ventricle	6,754	110	--	1,334	12,573	20,772
Cleft lip or palate	10,639	2,217	371	28,147	44,979	86,352
TE fistula	6,743	--	--	--	13,068	19,811
Atresia, small intestine	6,919	--	--	--	5,925	12,843
Colorectal atresia	6,267	--	--	--	20,470	26,737
Renal agenesis	2,707	--	--	--	50,458	53,165
Urinary obstruction	5,072	--	--	--	37,508	42,579
Upper-limb reduction	1,220	3,067	--	5,565	11,441	21,292
Lower-limb reduction	1,814	1,497	--	9,996	7,520	20,826
Diaphragmatic hernia	6,876	--	--	--	38,095	44,971
Gastroschisis	5,972	--	--	--	6,852	12,824

Table 7-2. (Continued)

Condition	Direct costs			Indirect costs		Total costs
	Medical (a)	Special education (b)	Developmental services (b)	Morbidity (c)	Mortality (c)	
Omphalocele	3,053	–	–	–	13,154	16,207
Down syndrome	30,528	37,133	12,004	95,541	53,525	228,731
Cerebral palsy	93,306	28,639	27,525	116,226	26,434	292,130

Note: Figures are based on lifetime direct and indirect cost estimates for the 1988 birth cohort in California. Costs beyond the first year of life were discounted back to the year of birth at a 5% discount rate, a rate commonly used in cost-of-illness studies. Row totals may not equal row sums because of rounding.

(a) Estimates of medical care costs are for care through the second year of life for conditions listed in quadrant I of Table 2-2 with the exception of colorectal atresia, for which estimates are through age seventeen. Congenital urinary tract obstruction may be associated with medical costs beyond the second year, but data limitations prevented estimation of such costs. For conditions listed in other quadrants of Table 2-2, estimates reflect costs through age sixty-five.

(b) Estimates are provided only for conditions for which there was an expectation of above-average rates of disability (those listed in quadrants II and IV of Table 2-2). Data limitations prevented us from estimating developmental and special education services costs associated with renal agenesis and developmental services costs associated with heart anomalies and limb reductions.

Table 7-3. Total cost of individual birth defects and aggregate costs, United States (a)

Condition	Total cost, 1988 ($1,000s)	Total cost, 1992 ($1,000s)	Total nonduplicative costs, 1992 ($1,000s) (b)
Spina bifida	388,990	489,289	489,289
Truncus arteriosus	164,465	209,676	175,919
Transposition/DORV	414,505	514,529	430,661
Tetralogy of Fallot	282,738	360,486	300,645
Single ventricle	148,417	172,631	149,671
Cleft lip or palate	575,419	696,501	625,458
TE fistula	132,007	165,002	128,867
Atresia, small intestine	85,581	110,061	63,835
Colorectal atresia	178,166	219,262	127,830
Renal agenesis	354,273	424,159	391,075
Urinary obstruction	283,731	343,223	329,151
Upper-limb reduction	141,882	170,036	132,288
Lower-limb reduction	138,777	167,067	130,479
Diaphragmatic hernia	299,671	364,348	331,192
Gastroschisis	85,453	108,763	87,228
Omphalocele	107,998	132,004	106,131
Down syndrome	1,524,182	1,847,752	1,847,752
Cerebral palsy	1,946,650	2,425,781	2,183,203
Total	N/A	N/A	8,030,672

(a) Figures reflect lifetime direct and indirect costs associated with birth defects for the cohort born with those conditions in 1988 discounted back to the year of birth at a 5% discount rate.

(b) Multiple cases of birth defects were assigned to one birth defect category as described in the text. Column total may not equal column sum because of rounding.

index.[b] The remainder of each estimate was inflated based on the increase in the employment cost index for civilian workers from the US Bureau of Labor Statistics. The relative size of the resultant cost estimates in column 2 of Table 7-3 reveals a similar pattern to that in California, ranging from $110 million for atresia of the small intestine to more than $2.4 billion for cerebral palsy.

An Aggregate Estimate

Researchers and policy-makers may be interested in the combined cost of all of the defects we estimated. We use such an aggregate estimate below, for example, in comparing our cost estimates to those of Rice et al.[2] in their aggregate cost-of-illness study. Because some infants are born with more than one of the birth defects we analyzed, however, summing our total cost estimates across defects would entail some double-counting. Based on a special analysis performed by the California Birth Defects Monitoring System (CBDMP) of all births in its ascertainment area between 1983 and 1988, we were able to estimate the extent to which infants were born with more than one of seventeen of the eighteen birth defects analyzed. The CBDMP data did not include cerebral palsy. Based on these data, the presence of multiple congenital anomalies of interest was relatively small (column 1 of Table 7-4). Approximately 90% of infants were born with a single condition of interest. Among the remaining 10%, the large majority was born with just one additional condition. In a few instances, however, infants were born with as many as five of the conditions we analyzed.[c] We assumed that the rate at which children were born with cerebral palsy and at least one other birth condition

---

[b]The medical care component of the 1988 national estimates provided in column 1 of Table 7-3 was estimated for each defect using the California proportion of medical care costs to total costs in Table 7-2.

[c]Multiple cases were taken from a cross-listing of ten categories among the seventeen defects: spina bifida; all four conotruncal heart defects; cleft lip or palate; tracheoesophageal fistula; intestinal atresia such as atresia of the small intestine and colorectal/anal atresia; kidney such as renal agenesis and urinary obstruction; limb reduction such as upper-limb reduction and lower-limb reduction; congenital diaphragmatic hernia; gastroschisis/omphalocele; and Down syndrome. Within-category multiple cases were ignored; thus, the resulting estimate may be slightly upward biased.

of interest was the average rate for all other defects.

In order to make an aggregate cost estimate that avoided double-counting, we assigned all multiple cases to the single-defect category among the multiple having the highest estimated average cost per case, as reported in Table 7-1.[d] We thereby assumed that an infant born with multiple defects would generate at least the average cost associated with the most expensive defect among the multiple. As an illustration, we assigned an individual born with spina bifida and cleft lip or palate to the category of spina bifida only and assumed that such an individual would generate at least the average incremental cost of spina bifida. This illustration is a conservative assumption because multiple defects generally entail above-average service requirements and work limitations.[e] The assignation of multiple cases in this fashion resulted in the reduction of the number of incident cases for several defects.[f] The number of unique incident cases by defect after the assignment of each case to a single defect category is listed in column 2 of Table 7-4. Those defects with relatively low costs per case and relatively high rates of associated anomalies experienced the greatest number of reductions in incident cases. Rather than 944 incident cases with cleft lip/palate, for example, the assignation to a single category of those with cleft lip/palate and other defects left 848 incident cases of cleft lip/palate. These nonduplicative cases multiplied by the cost per case (reprinted in column 3 of Table 7-4) yielded total nonduplicative costs reported in column 4 of Table 7-4. The estimated 1988 aggregate cost of this set of birth defects in California was $978.3 million.

----

[d]Under our methodology for assigning multiple defects, no cases of cerebral palsy would have been assigned to another category because the cost per case of cerebral palsy is the highest among all of the birth defects. The amount we subtracted because of a 10% multiple defect rate for those with cerebral palsy is, therefore, greater than the amount that would have been subtracted had we had actual data on the degree to which children with cerebral palsy had multiple conditions.

[e]On the other hand, the average cost of the defect category from which the case is withdrawn is likely to be slightly higher than it would have been had the average cost been constructed without the case that is now exclusively assigned to a different category.

[f]See Table 3-1 for the number of incident cases by birth defect category.

Table 7-4.   Aggregate cost of eighteen birth defects in California discounted at 5%

Condition	Nonmultiple cases as a percentage of incident cases	Nonmultiple incident cases (a), 1988	Cost per case, 1988 (b) ($1,000s)	Total cost, 1988 ($1,000s)
		(A)	(B)	(A x B)
Spina bifida	100.0	226	258	58,308
Truncus arteriosus	83.9	47	437	20,539
Transposition/DORV	83.7	220	237	52,140
Tetralogy of Fallot	83.4	156	227	35,412
Single ventricle	86.7	58	304	17,632
Cleft lip or palate	89.8	848	91	77,168
TE fistula	78.1	121	128	15,488
Atresia, small intestine	58.0	116	64	7,424
Colorectal atresia	58.3	141	110	15,510
Renal agenesis	92.2	213	230	48,990
Urinary obstruction	95.9	532	77	40,964
Upper-limb reduction	77.8	182	91	16,562
Lower-limb reduction	78.1	89	182	16,198
Diaphragmatic hernia	90.9	180	227	40,860
Gastroschisis	80.2	109	94	10,246
Omphalocele	80.4	82	159	13,038
Down syndrome	100.0	558	410	228,780
Cerebral palsy	90.0	591	445	262,995
Total (California)	88.9	4,469	219	978,254

(a) Multiple cases of birth defects were assigned to one birth defect category as described in the text.

(b) From Table 7-1, column 5.

The estimated aggregate cost for the nation in 1992 dollars is reported in column 3 of Table 7-3. The figures in this column are simply the proportions of nonduplicative cases (column 1 of Table 7-4) multiplied by the estimated total cost of each birth defect (column 2 of Table 7-3). The estimated aggregate cost of these eighteen

defects for the United States was $8.0 billion in 1992 dollars. Costs
at 2% and 10% discount rates, reported in Table 1-1, were $19.5
billion and $3.2 billion, respectively. Cost per case in 1992 dollars, by
discount rate, also were provided in Table 1-1.

Comparison With Other Estimates

In order to put our estimates into perspective, it is worthwhile to
compare them to earlier work. How does our aggregate cost
estimates compare, for example, to the $6.2 billion national cost
estimates of a group of congenital anomalies by Rice et al.[3] Are our
estimates higher or lower than previous estimates of individual birth
defects such as cerebral palsy and spina bifida?

An Earlier Aggregate Estimate

The analysis of Rice et al.[4] was a national study that included a
category of all congenital anomalies (more than 200) within a
specified range of ICD-9 codes (740-759) under a prevalence
approach, whereas we estimated the cost of eighteen selected birth
defects in a California cohort using an incidence approach.[g] Because
we analyzed far fewer defects, our cost estimates would certainly tend
to be lower. Because costs are more heavily discounted under the
incidence approach that we adopted, our estimates would also tend
to be lower than under the prevalence methodology adopted in the
earlier study. Ignoring the large difference in number of defects and
the differential impact of discounting implicit in the methodologies
between the two studies, we made several other adjustments to our
estimates, as described below, to facilitate a direct comparison and
to place our estimate into perspective relative to that of the other
study.
We made this comparison based on our 1988 cost estimates.
Because the Rice et al.[5] study discounted productivity losses due to
mortality at 4%, we recalculated all of our estimates at that rate. We
calculated a national aggregate estimate, as reported above, but

---

[g]See Chapter 2 for a detailed discussion of the differences between these two
approaches.

subtracted the nonduplicative cost of cerebral palsy, which was not included in the Rice et al. study. The projected 1988 aggregate cost of these birth defects in the United States, based upon these adjustments, was $6.3 billion.

The $6.2 billion Rice et al.[6] estimate of the national cost of congenital anomalies was expressed in 1980 prices. These estimates had to be adjusted to 1988 prices for purposes of comparison. We inflated the direct-cost component from this study, which is exclusively medical costs, by the increase in the medical care component of the consumer price index between 1980 and 1988 and the indirect cost component by the increase in average employee compensation from the US Bureau of Labor Statistics. The resultant estimate of costs in 1988 was $9.9 billion.

The national cost estimate of $6.3 billion projected from our study is for seventeen birth defects, whereas the inflation-adjusted $9.9 billion estimate from the study by Rice et al.[7] is for more than 200. Under the prevalence approach adopted by the Rice et al. study, costs are not discounted as heavily as under the incidence approach we adopted. For both reasons, one would expect that our cost estimate would be lower, perhaps by as much as an order of magnitude, given the disparity in the number of defects included in the two studies. The fact that our estimate for the cost of seventeen defects instead equals approximately two thirds of the estimate from the other study suggests that the societal costs of all birth defects likely exceed the Rice et al. estimate by a wide margin.

Several important factors appear to be critical in the differences pointed up by this comparison of estimated cost. First, our estimates of indirect mortality costs exceed our direct medical care cost estimates by nearly twice the ratio of the earlier study, despite the greater deflation of such indirect costs from discounting all lost productivity back to birth in our analysis. It is likely that many deaths experienced by those with birth defects, especially those subsequent to infancy, are attributed solely to other, perhaps more proximate, causes in the study by Rice et al.[8] even though congenital birth defects were likely an important underlying cause.[h] Data from CBDMP that we used in our study also suggested that deaths related

---

[h]See Chapter 2 for a more detailed discussion of this problem of attribution in the presence of associated anomalies in cost-of-illness methodology.

to birth defects are underreported on death certificate data such as that used in the aggregate study. Studies that rely on death certificate data will, therefore, tend to underestimate indirect mortality costs associated with birth defects. Second, we uncovered extensive indirect morbidity costs due to work limitations that for several defects exceeded direct medical care costs, whereas the Rice et al. study found such costs to be insignificant. Finally, the substantial nonmedical direct costs for developmental and special education services that we identified for certain birth defect categories should remind us that cost-of-illness investigators should not neglect such costs.

A Recent Cerebral Palsy Study

Surprisingly few studies have made estimates of the cost of individual birth defects. In a recent study sponsored by the National Foundation for Brain Research (NFBR),[9] the cost of cerebral palsy was estimated at $1.24 billion in 1991, utilizing a prevalence approach. In terms of methods and data, the study was very similar to the approach undertaken by Rice et al.[10] in their aggregate analysis. Medical expenditures were based on average expenditure per unit of service multiplied by estimates of the quantity of services provided. These per-unit estimates of cost were not specific to cerebral palsy.

Unlike the aggregate Rice et al.[11] estimate, however, cost estimates were not made strictly on the basis of the primary diagnosis in the study sponsored by the NFBR. Direct medical cost estimates were made for cerebral palsy appearing as the first through fifth diagnosis for inpatient stays ($318.2 million) and for the first through third diagnosis for physician visits ($49.0 million) for a total of $367.2 million. Indirect cost estimates ($870 million) were based on reported family income on the 1989 National Health Interview Survey (NHIS) relative to average family income reported on the Current Population Survey. These estimates, therefore, purported to capture all lost income of caregivers in the household, not strictly the lost earnings of the individual with cerebral palsy.

Our estimate of direct medical costs of cerebral palsy, excluding long-term care costs, which was not incorporated into the NFBR study, was $20.1 million for California in 1988 at a 5% discount rate. Adjusting this cost figure to the nation, based on differences in the number of births and cost differences between California and the United States, as above, and inflating it to 1991, based on the medical care component of the consumer price index, yielded $172 million. The NFBR estimate is $146 million higher.

This discrepancy is likely attributable, for the most part, to two factors. First, the difference in the use of discounting between the incidence and prevalence approaches is critical. As demonstrated in Chapter 4, medical care to treat cerebral palsy is not concentrated in infancy but continues throughout life. Under the incidence approach that we adopted, discounting of such costs reduces the estimated costs considerably relative to the prevalence approach undertaken by the NFBR study, for which direct medical costs among the prevalent population are not discounted. With a discount rate of 2% rather than 5%, for example, our 1991 estimate of medical costs related to cerebral palsy would be $282 million, more than $100 million higher than at a 5% rate. Second, we subtracted medical care costs of the average person from our estimates in order to calculate incremental costs, whereas the NFBR study assumed that all hospital stays and visits in which cerebral palsy appeared as a contributing diagnosis constituted care above and beyond that experienced by the "average" person. It is likely that cerebral palsy is perceived by the provider as a contributing factor to nearly any medical care stay or visit, however, for someone with the disease. Had we not subtracted average costs, our 1991 estimate of such medical costs for cerebral palsy, at a 5% discount rate, would have been $330 million, which is much closer to the NFBR estimate. At a 2% rate, our estimate would have exceeded the NFBR estimate.[i]

Other factors also may have contributed to the difference. Our deflation of inpatient charges by the Medicare charge-to-cost ratio, for example, may have contributed to a lower medical care cost estimate because commercial insurers, on average, pay more than the Medicare allowance for inpatient services. Our use of financial data related to actual episodes of care for those with the illness, whereas relying on gross averages across all care also added precision to our estimates, which might be a factor in the discrepancy.

---

[i]We should note, however, that our estimate includes a projection for inpatient medical care episodes in which cerebral palsy was not listed as a contributing diagnosis (Table 4-1). The NFBR study did not include the cost of such episodes.

The NFBR study did not estimate the indirect mortality costs of cerebral palsy. Its estimate of $870 million in indirect morbidity costs, however, includes an estimate of lost income of family members. This NFBR estimate is for the prevalent population in one year only. By comparison, our estimate of indirect morbidity costs of cerebral palsy projected to the nation is $924.8 million at a 5% discount rate. The fact that we did not include lost income of family members suggests that our estimate should be lower. Instead, it is more than $50 million higher than the NFBR estimate. Part of this difference is likely attributable to the fact that our estimate includes lost compensation and not simply earnings; compensation includes fringe benefits. Furthermore, our figures incorporate an imputed value of household production, whereas the NFBR study did not. Finally, we estimated all such lost productivity over the entire life span for the cohort born with the disease in 1988, whereas the NFBR study estimated such costs for one year among the entire prevalent population with cerebral palsy. The cost of future productivity was heavily discounted under our methodology, however, whereas no discounting was performed under the prevalence approach adopted in the NFBR study.

An unlikely source of any major discrepancy between the two studies should arise from prevalence estimates of cerebral palsy because the National Health Interview Survey (NHIS) provided the basis for such estimates in both cases. However, the NFBR study used only one year of NHIS data (1989), whereas we made use of five years of pooled data (1985-1989).[j] These data permitted greater precision in terms of estimating prevalence and, hence, cost.

The differences in the estimates of common components between the two studies is of some interest, but the considerable costs related to components that the NFBR did not estimate are of much greater import. Our estimated cost of long-term care for those with cerebral palsy was approximately three times the cost of other direct medical care, for example. The direct cost of developmental services and special education combined were more than double the cost of direct medical care, and the indirect mortality costs associated with cerebral palsy also was substantial. Consequently, the total cost of cerebral

---

[j]See Chapter 3 for a discussion of prevalence estimates. A description of the NHIS is provided in Appendix 2.

palsy in our study projected to the nation in 1991 was $2.3 billion, nearly double the NFBR estimate. This large difference is due primarily to cost categories ignored by the NFBR study rather than to underlying discrepancies in estimates between common components.

A Recent Spina Bifida Study

Lipscomb[12] used an incidence approach to estimate the cost effectiveness of screening to prevent neural tube defects (NTDs) such as spina bifida. The author estimated the cost of spina bifida in North Carolina in 1985 for three different levels of lesions: thoracic or high lumbar, low lumbar, and sacral. Medical costs were estimated based on the examination of clinical records of 103 spina bifida victims treated at two North Carolina hospitals. Other nonmedical direct costs such as home modification expenses were made based on 112 responses to a survey conducted by the North Carolina Spina Bifida Association of member families. Additional cost estimates, based mainly on secondary data sources, were made of institutionalized care for spina bifida victims with mental retardation, developmental services, and special education, as well as for other services such as foster care. Based on responses to the above questionnaire, an estimate also was made of lost parental income because of home care of the victim. An estimate of total costs for the "modal case" of spina bifida in North Carolina, discounted at 5%, was $181,745 (1985 dollars).[k]

We demonstrated in Chapter 4 that the Lipscomb[13] estimates for medical care for open spina bifida victims, by age group, bear a striking similarity to our own. Adjustment of the remaining costs for price changes between 1985 and 1988 leaves the estimate from the Lipscomb study close to our estimate of $234,000 per case (in 1988 dollars, adjusted to the nation), even though Lipscomb included an estimate of parental productivity loss not incorporated in our study, as well as a higher rate of institutionalization for mentally retarded spina bifida victims. Our use of a more refined methodology, coupled with primary data sources for calculating special education

---

[k]This estimate includes the assumption of 100% "replacement," which is analogous in our study to subtracting the costs associated with the average child.

and productivity loss because of heightened morbidity from spina
bifida, resulted in substantially higher estimates for these components,
which produced final estimates comparable to those of Lipscomb.

Strengths and Limitations

Our research represents the first attempt to apply cost-of-illness
methodology to a wide array of several of the most clinically
significant structural birth defects among the general population. The
incidence approach undertaken in the book was strengthened by
newly released population data from the CBDMP, one of the most
extensive active surveillance efforts with respect to birth defects in the
world.

Certain aspects of our methodology make our results conservative.
We did not estimate the indirect cost to society, for example, due to
parents and other family members who take time from work to care
for those with chronic disabilities because of birth defects. Such costs
can be substantial. As mentioned earlier, Lipscomb[14] estimated that
the net average annual reduction in parental income averaged $7,195
in 1985 dollars for children aged zero to nine with open spina bifida
and $8,362 for such children aged ten to seventeen. Psychosocial
costs (the pain and suffering of individuals with birth defects or their
families) also were not estimated, although they may exceed
traditional human capital costs.[15]

We may have underestimated disability rates and, hence, indirect
morbidity costs for certain defects because the data set from which
we estimated work limitations (NHIS) excludes institutionalized
persons (Appendix 2). We also may have underestimated
developmental services costs for some conditions because the
Department of Developmental Services (DDS) file (Appendix 2)
included only public expenditures and excluded private, out-of-pocket
spending for services such as special vehicles, transportation, home
modification, and appliances. Studies conducted by the United
Cerebral Palsy Association found that average cerebral palsy-related
expenses for families with children with cerebral palsy ranged from
$6,994 to $10,059 (1991 dollars).[16]

Because of the underlying structure of the DDS file, it is likely that
we even underestimated public expenditures on developmental

services for conditions other than cerebral palsy. Among the conditions we analyzed, cerebral palsy is the lone "qualifying condition" for services from the DDS. Reporting of conditions other than a "qualifying condition" on the DDS file is contingent on accurate recording of "underlying etiologies" and "contributing conditions." Developmental costs may be underestimated because of the recent incorporation of ICD-9 codes for underlying etiologies on the DDS file in 1984 and because certain conditions such as cleft lip may not always be considered a significant contributor to developmental service requirements.

Our decision to estimate incremental medical care costs only through age one for conditions listed in quadrant I of Table 2-2 was based on the available medical literature, as was our decision to estimate lifetime mortality costs for conditions in quadrants I and II based on infant mortality only. These decisions also were partly driven by constraints imposed by available data. To the extent that excess medical care services are provided past age one and premature mortality continues past infancy, we underestimated the associated costs.

It is traditional that cost-of-illness studies utilize administrative data in order to make medical and other incremental cost estimates based strictly on the presence of the diagnosis of interest on the record of each unit of service such as physician visit, a hospital stay, or a prescription. However, as discussed in Chapter 2, this procedure may ignore services rendered for conditions or circumstances that seemed to the provider to be so remote to the underlying birth defect that the condition was not recorded as a contributing diagnosis, even though a positive association may exist from a population perspective. Even though a birth defect may be associated with heightened susceptibility to infection or accidents for several years subsequent to surgical repair, the specific provider who treats such infection or injury may be unaware of the existence of the defect. For these reasons, we attempted to calculate all services rendered to individuals with birth defects and to estimate incremental costs by subtracting such services normally provided within the general population. Absent comprehensive longitudinal data on services provided to those with birth defects, however, we invariably underestimated the total amount of such services provided. An illustration of the extent to which services may go unreported from the absence of longitudinal data was illustrated by our adjustment of medical costs in Chapter 4 based on the comparison of data from the MediCal claims file, which has a one-year longitudinal component, to individual hospital abstract data from the Office of Statewide Health Planning and Development in California (OSHPD). Still more comprehensive longitudinal data likely would have increased our estimates of cost.

We estimated a lifetime profile of direct and indirect costs based on a cross-sectional profile of norms of disability, treatment, and earnings in and around 1988. To the extent that new medical care technologies or new policies regarding special education and employment of those with disabilities make future patterns of care more costly, we underestimated costs. Of course, new technologies and policies also could reduce the costs of such treatment and care.

Cost as the Foundation for Assessing Interventions

The cost estimates provided in this study provide the basis for assessing a prevention strategy in cost-benefit analysis or comparing competing strategies with respect to a single birth defect or across several birth defects in cost-effectiveness analyses. The estimated cost per case listed by condition in Table 1-1 is the average societal benefit that one would expect in the United States from preventing a single case of each birth defect. Recent findings that folate supplementation may reduce the risk of NTDs, such as spina bifida, and provide the impetus to undertake a detailed cost-benefit analysis of a program to fortify foods with folate using estimates from our study of costs. This analysis, reported below, provides an example of how our cost estimates can inform policy.

A Cost/Benefit Analysis of Folate Fortification to Prevent Neural Tube Defects[1,17]

A program that lowers the incidence of NTDs could produce substantial economic benefits. Several observational studies and randomized trials have suggested that periconceptional folic acid supplementation reduces the risk of NTDs,[18,19] even among women

---

[1]The analysis presented in this section draws heavily on Romano, Waitzman, Scheffler, and Pi (endnote 17).

without a previously affected pregnancy.[20,21,22] In response, the US Public Health Service recommended in September 1992 that "all women of childbearing age . . . who are capable of becoming pregnant should consume 0.4 mg of folic acid per day for the purpose of reducing their risk of having a pregnancy affected by . . . NTDs."[23]

Three approaches to implementing this recommendation include increasing dietary folate intake by promoting consumption of fresh vegetables and legumes, fortifying staple foods, and increasing consumption of folic acid supplements.[24] Food fortification offers several advantages over the other approaches. Because the neural tube closes during the fourth week of gestation, folate must be provided before many women realize that they are pregnant. Yet more than half of all pregnancies in the United States are unplanned[25] and 13.2 million sexually active women of child-bearing age are not using effective contraception.[26] Because fortification does not require behavior modification, it would reach more of this target population. For these reasons, the Food and Drug Administration (FDA) recently proposed amending the standards of identity for enriched grain products to include folic acid.[27]

Cost-benefit analysis provides a structured framework for comparing anticipated costs and benefits; thus, strategies likely to produce net benefits can be identified. In the present analysis, we focused on the proposed fortification of grain with folic acid but considered dietary supplements as an alternative. Our analysis has been described in detail elsewhere but will be summarized here.[28]

Analytic framework and level of fortification — The economic benefit of fortification equals the product of the incremental cost associated with each NTD case and the number of cases averted. Our estimate of the latter quantity is based on estimates of how many more women in the target population would consume adequate folate if fortification was instituted and how much an individual' s risk of having an affected child would be reduced. The economic cost of fortification includes costs related to food production and adverse health effects. The impact of altering key assumptions was tested using sensitivity analysis.

All of our estimates are based on two fortification strategies, which were selected from a list of fourteen presented to the FDA' s Folic Acid Subcommittee in April 1993.[29] These low and high strategies involve fortification of enriched cereal grains with folic acid at 140 mcg (twice that necessary to replace milling losses) or 350 mcg (five times the replacement level) per 100 g. Cereal grains include flours made from wheat, rice, barley, triticale, buckwheat, corn, or rye; corn meal or grits; rice; farina; and macaroni or pasta. Cereal grains are an obvious candidate for fortification because they are consumed by most women of child-bearing age and are already subject to standards of identity for nutrient enrichment. These standards require millers who enrich their products to use a standard formula that generally includes thiamine, riboflavin, niacin, and iron.[30]

Estimating costs: food production — Pure folic acid was available to food processors at a 1991 price of $115 per kilogram (T Viespoli, telephone communication, August 1993). In order to estimate the cost of fortifying each unit of grain, an "overage" factor of 1.3 was applied to reflect the additional folic acid that food processors would buy to compensate for losses during grain storage, baking, packaging, and shipment (H Gordon, telephone communication, July 1993).

Under these assumptions, the unit cost of folic acid fortification would be $.0095 per 100 pounds of grain at 140 mcg/100 g and $.0237 per 100 pounds of grain at 350 mcg/100 g. Total direct costs were estimated by multiplying these unit costs by "domestic food disappearance" in 1991 (US Department of Agriculture, unpublished data, July 1993), adjusted downward to exclude the unenriched portion that would not be fortified (Table 7-5).[31,32] Domestic disappearance is a measure of human consumption; it represents the difference between total supply (domestic production plus imports and stocks on August 1, 1990) and other uses (exports, animal feed, nonfood uses, and stocks on August 1, 1991). We assumed that folic acid would not be added to grain destined for export, animal feed, or nonfood uses or to grains that lack standards of identity.

Folic acid fortification limited to currently enriched grains would not require additional equipment. Analytic testing to confirm appropriate folate levels was estimated to cost $2.5 million annually.[33] Changing product labels would involve a one-time cost of $50 to $500 per package or $20 million nationwide[34] ($1.0 million annually, assuming perpetual yield at a 5% discount rate). Fortification with folic acid does not affect the appearance, taste, or shelf life of cooked corn meal,[35] wheat bread,[36] or wine.[37] We therefore assumed that fortification would have no other production-

Table 7-5. Total direct costs associated with universal fortification of cereal grains in the United States with two levels of folic acid (1991$)

Cereal grain	Total domestic disappearance, million hundred (lbs.) (a)	Currently enriched (%) (b)	Cost: folic acid ($ x 10⁶) (c)		Other costs: ($ x 10⁶) (d)		Cost: total ($ x 10⁶)	
			Low level	High level	Low level	High level	Low level	High level
Wheat flour (e)	344.855	90	2.95	7.37				
Rice (f)	42.300	90 White / 00 Brown	0.27	0.69				
Corn flour/meal	35.600	10	0.03	0.08				
Corn hominy/grits	8.600	01	0.00	0.00				
Total (g)	433.320	80	3.26	8.14	24.88	41.26	28.14	49.40

(a) From the US Department of Agriculture's Economic Research Service (J Putnam, written communication, July 1993). Methods are described by Putnam and Allshouse.

(b) Assumes an incremental unit cost of $.0095 per 100 pounds of grain for low-level fortification (140 mcg folate/100 g) and $.0237 per 100 pounds of grain for high-level fortification (350 mcg folate/100 g), including 30% overage to compensate for losses during packaging, storage, and shipment. These costs are adjusted downward to reflect the proportion of domestic production that is currently enriched (and would, therefore, be subject to the proposed standards of identity).

(c) From written and telephone communications in July 1993 with R Henwood (Millers National Federation), J Scesland (Milling and Baking News), W Goldsmith (USA Rice Council), M Androus (CA Rice Promotion Board), D Salomen (Lauhoff Grain Company), S Rao (CONAGRA), and J Otwell (Cook Flour Company). The current standard of identity for enriched cereal grains does not include folic acid.

(d) Other annual costs include $2.5 million for analytical testing; $0.8 million for label changes (perpetual yield of a $20 million capitalized asset, with a 5% discount rate); $16.4 million (low level) or $32.8 million (high level) for direct and indirect costs of neurologic sequelae among patients with undiagnosed vitamin B₁₂ deficiency; and $5 million for surveillance of these sequelae. (Chapter 3 provides a discussion of prevalence estimates, and a description of the NHIS is provided in Appendix 2.)

(e) Includes white flour, whole wheat flour, durum or semolina flour (8%), and farina.

(f) Includes white rice (76%) and brown rice (24%). Note that substantial (20% to 100%) nutrient loss occurs if consumers wash rice fortified by the inexpensive "powder" method, which is used in at least half of domestically enriched rice (K Hargrove, Rice Millers Association), as described by Hoffpauer.

(g) Excludes flour derived from rye, rice, barley, buckwheat, or triticale because these grain products are not subject to a standard of identity for enrichment.

related costs.

Estimating costs: adverse health effects — The adverse health effects of folic acid fortification are difficult to estimate. Folate-containing supplements administered to pregnant women have no long-term developmental, behavioral, or neurologic effects on children resulting from these pregnancies.[38] Folic acid is very safe when administered to healthy subjects.[39] However, there is concern about adverse health effects among persons taking anticonvulsant or antifolate medications and persons with undiagnosed pernicious anemia.

Several anticonvulsants, including phenytoin and phenobarbital, affect folate metabolism. In animal models, folates activate epileptic foci and impair the ability of phenobarbital to raise the seizure threshold.[40,41,42] Folic acid supplements also lower serum phenytoin levels.[43,44] However, numerous controlled trials have found no effect of oral folic acid on seizure control at doses up to 20 mg daily.[45,46,47,48,49,50,51,52,53,54] Other commonly used medications with antifolate effects include methotrexate, pyrimethamine, trimethoprim, triamterene, and sulfasalazine. Folic acid does not reduce the therapeutic effectiveness of methotrexate in rheumatoid arthritis.[55,56] Adverse drug interactions involving dietary folate are conceivable but could be avoided at minimal expense through educational efforts such as drug labels, package inserts, and professional publications.

The most worrisome effect of folic acid is its ability to induce remission of megaloblastic anemia due to vitamin B_{12} deficiency[57] while neurologic manifestations progress. Daily doses of 300 to 500 mcg may induce partial remission,[58,59,60,61,62] but doses of at least 1 mg are generally required for complete remission[63,64,65] and relapses are frequent.[66] Since 1947, at least 80 patients with vitamin B_{12} deficiency have developed subacute combined degeneration (SCD) of the spinal cord or other neurologic sequelae despite hematologic improvement on folic acid.[67,68,69,70,71,72,73,74,75,76,77,78,79] Prompt administration of vitamin B_{12} improved neurologic symptoms in most, but not all, patients.

Based on limited data, we estimated the number of additional cases of neurologic disease likely to result from folate fortification, as well as the associated costs. Two European studies have reported the annual incidence of diagnosed pernicious anemia (without fortification) as 9.5[80] to 16.7[81] per 100,000 persons. The higher estimate corresponds to 38,000 new cases in the United States in 1991. With low-level or high-level fortification, 5% or 10%, respectively, of these patients would have received enough folate to mask the anemia that led to their diagnosis (assuming a threshold of 0.85 mg/day). Approximately 24% to 26% of these responders would have been expected to develop neurologic signs.[82] Therefore, folate fortification in 1991 would have allowed approximately 500 PA patients to develop neurologic disease.

We then posited that all of these neurologic sequelae would have been as costly as SCD and that each case would have required one hospitalization in 1991. According to the 1989 National Hospital Discharge Survey, the mean duration of hospitalization for patients with SCD or related disorders was sixteen days,[83] and the mean cost per day (inflated to 1991) was $867.[84] We applied a hospital-to-physician-services-cost ratio (specific to spinal cord diseases) of 4.7:1[85] and a multiplier of 1.83 (specific to elderly persons with neurologic disorders)[86] to reflect the additional cost of drugs, nursing home care, appliances, and other professional services. Indirect costs were approximately 6.4% of direct costs among elderly persons with neurologic disorders;[87] thus, the total cost of fortification-related neurologic disease was estimated at $16.4 million ($32,700 per case). This estimate may be too high because (a) many neurologic sequelae are less severe than SCD; (b) mild SCD does not require hospitalization; (c) the diagnosis and treatment of SCD may be delayed, thus, the costs may be paid with discounted dollars; and (d) vitamin B_{12} assays would detect many cases of masked PA at a reversible stage.[88] However, our estimate may be too low if severe SCD leads to late complications or lifelong skilled nursing care.

In light of the controversy surrounding the potential impact of folic acid fortification on the incidence of SCD, follow-up surveillance would be necessary. The incremental cost of this effort was estimated at $5 million ($1 to $10 million) (JD Erickson, telephone communication, August 1993).

Estimating benefits: reduction in the risk of neural tube defects—The literature on periconceptional folate and NTDs includes two randomized, controlled, double-blind trials[89,90] and three nonrandomized trials among women with a previous NTD pregnancy;[91,92,93,94] one randomized[95] and one nonrandomized[96] trial among women without such a history; six case control studies,[97,98,99,100,101,102,103] and one cohort study.[104] All but one[105] of these studies suggested a favorable effect of dietary or supplemental folate. The effectiveness of dietary fortification is difficult to estimate because none of the randomized trials used fortification, yet the bioavailability of folic acid in foodstuffs is 50% to 60% of that in liquid[106] or tablet[107] form. However, all four studies that explored the NTD-diet association[108,109,110,111] are consistent with the Medical Research Council's finding of 67% effectiveness.[112] We used the Centers for Disease Control's estimate of 50% effectiveness, with literature-based sensitivity limits of 67% and 20%.[113]

The daily intake of dietary folate necessary to achieve this benefit may be as low as 100 mcg;[114] however, two case-control studies show a graded dose-response relationship up to 311[115] or 350 mcg[116] daily. We conservatively assumed a target level of 400 mcg, which equals the proposed recommended daily allowance for pregnant or lactating women.[117] A target level of 200 mcg was tested in a sensitivity analysis.[118,119]

Estimating benefits: baseline folate intake—Folic acid currently is added to a limited number of foods in the United States, such as breakfast cereals and diet supplements.[120] Despite voluntary efforts,[121] only 8% or less of adult women obtained 400 mcg of dietary folate daily in 1976-1980[122] and 1985-1986.[123] More recent data from 1988-1991 suggest little improvement.[124] In the 1986 NHIS, 27% of nonpregnant women aged eighteen to forty-four years used a folate-containing supplement at least once during the preceding two weeks.[125] Several population-based studies confirm these estimates, with 12% to 15% of women regularly supplemented and 7% to 9%[126,127] partially supplemented during the periconceptional period.[128,129,130]

Our best estimate of the percentage of women in the target population already receiving sufficient folate to minimize the risk of an NTD is 33% (27% from supplements, 8% from diet, and 2% from both). For sensitivity analysis, this percentage could be as low as 13% or as high as 40%, if supplement use has increased since 1987. If the threshold for lowering NTD risk is 200 mcg rather than 400 mcg, then 56% of the target population is receiving adequate folate

(27% from supplements, 40% from diet, and 11% from both).

Estimating benefits: effect of fortification on folate intake—According to the FDA' s analysis of data from the 1987-1988 Nationwide Food Consumption Survey, grain fortification at 140 mcg per 100 g would enable approximately 50% of women aged eleven to fifty years to receive at least 400 mcg of folate daily.[131] Grain fortification at 350 mcg per 100 g would enable approximately 75% of these women to receive the desired amount of folate. The portion of the target population that would begin consuming adequate folate after fortification would be 17% (50% to 33%) with low-level and 42% (75% to 33%) with high-level fortification. Even though actual food intake is 18% to 30% higher than that reported in consumption surveys,[132,133] approximately 20% of domestic cereal grain production is unenriched. These effects almost cancel each other. If the threshold for lowering NTD risk is 200 mcg rather than 400 mcg, then the portion of the target population likely to benefit is 29% (85% to 56%) with low-level and 39% (95% to 56%) with high-level fortification.

Estimating benefits: value of preventing a neural tube defect—The benefit of preventing each NTD case equals the net present value of lifetime costs associated with a child in the 1991 birth cohort after subtracting the costs associated with an average child.[134] We assumed that if an NTD case had been prevented by adequate folate intake, the affected child would have been born with the baseline risk of other defects or illnesses. Because the unit of analysis was the individual, our estimates for spina bifida include the costs of associated anomalies and illnesses. Our best estimate incorporates a discount rate of 5%, even though we tested rates of 2% and 10% in sensitivity analyses.[m]

For anencephaly, incremental direct costs were assumed to be zero. Anencephaly is rapidly and uniformly fatal; thus, there are no outpatient, long-term care, developmental, or special education costs.

---

[m]This range of discount rates differs from the 2.5% to 6% range used in our previously published analysis. We adopted the 2% to 10% rates here so as to maintain consistency with the rates used to estimate figures throughout the rest of this volume.

There are also few morbidity costs; in fact, all anencephalic births incur the human capital costs associated with premature mortality.

Table 7-6 shows our final estimates of per capita costs for the average American child born with spina bifida or anencephaly in 1991. These estimates are based on our 1988 California estimates reported in Table 7-1 adjusted for cost differences between California and the nation, and for inflation between 1988 and 1991, as described earlier with respect to our construction of aggregate estimates.

Estimating benefits: other effects of fortification—Folates may improve perinatal outcomes independent of their effect on neural tube closure. Folic acid supplements raise mean birth weight in indigent populations,[135,136] but observational[137,138] and randomized studies[139,140,141,142] in well-nourished populations have produced inconsistent results. Even though some investigators have reported that multivitamins with folic acid prevent recurrences of facial clefts,[143,144,145] this conclusion was refuted by two randomized controlled trials.[146,147] Given conflicting evidence, we assumed that fortification would not affect the incidence of low birthweight or cleft deformities.

Folate deficiency may be a factor in carcinogenesis.[148] Even though a preliminary study of women with mild to moderate cervical dysplasia suggested that folic acid supplementation may induce regression,[149] this finding was not confirmed in a larger trial[150] and is not supported by epidemiologic data.[151,152,153] Patients with ulcerative colitis may lower their risk of colorectal cancer by consuming supplemental folic acid.[154] Folic acid with vitamin B_{12} may decrease host susceptibility to carcinogens,[155] but it is unclear whether fortification of grain would affect the incidence of cancer.

Finally, low-plasma-folate levels and folate-deficient diets have been linked to high homocysteine levels[156] that, in turn, are associated with increased risk of atherosclerosis.[157] Even though folate supplementation may reverse hyperhomocysteinemia,[158] its effect on atherosclerosis remains speculative.

Best estimate of net benefit—According to combined data from sixteen surveillance systems, the prevalence of spina bifida between 1983 and 1990 was 4.6 per 10,000 live births.[159] The birth prevalence of anencephaly is more difficult to ascertain because these infants are considered stillborn in some areas. The CBDMP reports

Table 7-6. Total incremental costs ($) associated with one case of spina bifida or anencephaly, United States, 1991

Condition/cost component	California, 1988 Discount rate			United States average, 1991 Discount rate		
	2%	5%	10%	2%	5%	10%
Spina bifida						
Medical care	127,659	99,124	73,341	147,798	114,761	84,911
Developmental services	1,636	993	610	1,703	1,034	635
Special education	30,805	23,261	15,278	32,062	24,210	15,901
Indirect: mortality cost	244,920	82,367	18,217	254,912	85,727	18,960
Indirect: morbidity cost	154,035	52,518	11,792	137,958	54,661	12,273
Total costs	559,102	258,296	121,266	574,433	280,393	132,680
Anencephaly						
Indirect: mortality cost	976,837	329,116	73,015	1,016,690	342,543	75,994
Total costs	976,837	329,116	73,015	1,016,690	342,543	75,994

that anencephaly occurs in 2.7 per 10,000 live births (T Bateson, written communication, July 1993).

Assuming that adequate folate intake lowers the risk of an NTD pregnancy by 50%, the target population can be separated into two subpopulations. Among the 33% who receive adequate folate ($\geq$ 400 mcg/day), the expected prevalence of spina bifida and anencephaly would be 2.7 and 1.6 per 10,000 live births, respectively. Among the 67% who receive inadequate folate, the expected prevalence of spina bifida and anencephaly would be twice as high or 5.5 and 3.2 per 10,000, respectively, live births. Low-level fortification of grain would shift 17% of the target population from high risk to low risk, whereas high-level fortification would shift 42% of the target population. With 4,111,000 live births in the United States in 1991,[160] low-level fortification would have averted 191 spina bifida cases and 113 anencephaly cases, and high-level fortification would have averted 473 spina bifida cases and 280 anencephaly cases.

The economic benefit from preventing these NTDs amounts to $92.3 million with low-level and $228.5 million with high-level fortification. These figures far exceed the costs of fortification shown in Table 7-5; the differences of $64.1 million (low level) and $179.2 million (high level) represent the net benefit of fortification. The estimated benefit-cost ratio is 3.3:1 for low-level and 4.6:1 for high-level fortification.

Sensitivity analysis — Table 7-7 shows the net economic benefit and the benefit-cost ratio computed under a range of assumptions about the discount rate, the baseline level of folate intake in the target population, the effectiveness of dietary folate in preventing NTDs, the threshold dose of folic acid that minimizes the risk of an affected child, and the cost of comprehensive surveillance. The benefit-cost ratio remains favorable with any plausible value of these variables.

Cost effectiveness compared with supplement use — Promoting voluntary use of folate supplements is another strategy to prevent NTDs. We could not estimate the net economic benefit of such a program because adherence is not predictable. The cost per NTD averted was estimated assuming that (a) all folate supplements have at least 400 mcg of folic acid; (b) all purchased supplements would be consumed; (c) only members of the target population would respond to public education; (d) no members of this population would develop neurologic sequelae of vitamin B_{12} deficiency; (e) excess consumption beyond 400 mcg daily would be negligible; and (f) supplement use would be independent of dietary folate intake. At a minimum annualized price of $12 ($3.29/100 tablets; Davis, California), United States consumers would spend $132,000 in order to avert each NTD case. The comparable cost per NTD averted would be $92,500 for low-level and $65,500 for high-level fortification (Table 7-7).

Summary of folate fortification analysis—This analysis shows that fortification of cereal grains in the United States with folic acid would probably have economic benefits that significantly exceed the costs. Even though high-level fortification might have greater net economic benefits and a larger cost-benefit ratio than low-level fortification, the latter strategy may be preferable in the short term because it poses little risk to persons with undiagnosed vitamin B_{12} deficiency. If future surveillance reveals no adverse consequences, the fortification level could be increased to reach a greater proportion of the target population. Of course, we may have underestimated net benefits because of unmeasured costs of NTDs (e.g., parental out-of-pocket expenses,[161] opportunity costs,[162,163,164,165,166,167,168] and pain and suffering) and unmeasured benefits of higher folate intake. Conversely, we have overestimated net benefits if the cost of neurologic sequelae related to delayed diagnosis of vitamin B_{12} deficiency exceeds our projection.

Other Interventions

Other interventions lend themselves to use cost-benefit analysis based on our estimates of birth defect costs. Fetal surgery for correction of life-threatening birth defects, for example, is another approach that can be evaluated using the cost figures in this book. Repair of congenital diaphragmatic hernia (CDH) in utero, for example, may allow normal lung growth during the last trimester of pregnancy and thereby obviate the need for expensive postnatal therapies such as extracorporeal membrane oxygenation.[169] The financial costs of fetal surgery and associated care, which averaged $10,400 among the first seventeen cases at the University of California, San Francisco,[170] may be substantially less than the cost

Table 7-7. Sensitivity analysis of the net economic benefit and the benefit-cost ratio associated with low-level and high-level fortification of cereal grains in the United States, 1991

Assumption/value assigned	Net economic benefit, $ x 10^6 (a)		Ratio of benefits to costs		Cost per case averted, $ x 10^3 (no. of cases)	
	Low level	High level	Low level	High level	Low level	High level
Discount rate						
2.0%	197.1	507.6	8.2	11.4	90.6 (304)	64.8 (753)
5.0% (best estimate) (b)	64.1	179.2	3.3	4.6	92.5 (304)	65.5 (753)
10.0%	4.8	33.7	1.2	1.7	95.7 (304)	66.8 (753)
Percentage of target population with adequate folate intake at baseline						
13%	151.5	251.6	6.4	6.1	47.5 (592)	49.8 (992)
33% (best estimate) (b)	64.1	179.2	3.3	4.6	92.5 (304)	65.5 (753)
40%	28.6	149.4	2.0	4.0	150.5 (187)	75.4 (655)
Reduction in NTD risk associated with adequate folate intake						
20%	4.6	32.2	1.2	1.7	260.6 (108)	183.6 (269)
50% (best estimate) (b)	64.1	179.2	3.3	4.6	92.5 (304)	65.5 (753)
67%	104.5	278.6	4.7	6.6	64.4 (437)	45.7 (1081)
Folate intake necessary to minimize NTD risk (threshold dose)						
200 mcg	154.9	196.4	6.5	5.0	46.7 (602)	61.0 (810)
400 mcg (best estimate) (b)	64.1	179.2	3.3	4.6	92.5 (304)	65.5 (753)

Table 7-7. (Continued)

Assumption/value assigned	Net economic benefit, $ x 10^6 (a)		Ratio of benefits to costs		Cost per case averted, $ x 10^3 (no. of cases)	
	Low level	High level	Low level	High level	Low level	High level
Cost of surveillance program						
$1 million	68.1	183.1	3.8	5.0	79.4 (304)	60.3 (753)
$5 million (best estimate) (b)	64.1	179.2	3.3	4.6	92.5 (304)	65.5 (753)
$10 million	59.1	174.1	2.8	4.2	109.0 (304)	72.2 (753)

(a) The net economic benefit represents the difference between total benefits and total costs, where:

$$TC \text{ (total cost)} = COST_{folate} + COST_{sdosing} + COST_{assays} + COST_{surveillance} + COST_{vitamin \, B12 \, deficiency}$$

$$TB \text{ (total benefit)} = \Sigma \, [(LB_{US}) * (ADEQ_{post} \cdot ADEQ_{prior}) * (NTDRATE_{inadeq} - NTDRATE_{adeq}) * PERCAP]$$

where LB_{US} is the total number of live births in the United States in 1991, $ADEQ_{post}$ and $ADEQ_{prior}$ are the proportions of the target population receiving enough folate to minimize the risk of an NTD after and before fortification, $NTDRATE_{inadeq}$ and $NTDRATE_{adeq}$ are hypothetical NTD incidence rates without and with adequate folate intake, and PERCAP is the lifetime total of direct and indirect costs associated with one NTD case born in 1991. This quantity is summed across NTDs (e.g., spina bifida plus anencephaly).

(b) The "best estimate" is based on the following assumptions: (a) a 5.0% discount rate, (b) 33% of the target population has adequate folate intake at baseline (from diet or vitamin supplements), (c) adequate folate intake reduces the risk of an NTD pregnancy by 50%, (d) the threshold daily dose of folate necessary to minimize the risk of an NTD pregnancy is 400 mcg, and (e) the cost of a surveillance program to monitor adverse effects is $5 million.

of a child born with CDH (estimated at $250,000 in 1992 dollars at a 5% discount rate). Fetal surgery also may be cost beneficial for congenital bilateral hydronephrosis because in utero repair may prevent serious renal injury and correct oligohydramnios (which is associated with pulmonary hypoplasia).[171] The economic benefits of preventing urinary tract anomalies should be considered in estimating the cost-benefit relationship for cocaine addiction treatment programs.[172] Intensive multidisciplinary treatment programs, which significantly reduce the incidence of congenital malformations in diabetic pregnancies,[173] are probably even more cost effective than is currently recognized.[174]

The Case for Additional Research

In spite of known strategies to prevent birth defects, our current state of knowledge regarding the etiology of birth defects is limited. Research is the first stage in the development of new prevention strategies. Yet, the annual national research effort supported by the major institutional funders in this area such as the National Institutes of Health, March of Dimes Birth Defects Foundation, Centers for Disease Control, and Shriner' s Hospitals was less than $100 million in 1992,[175] which is approximately one third the estimated annual national cost of special education for those born with Down syndrome in that year. This estimate of research effort incorporated a much broader definition of birth defects than the structural anomalies for which we studied costs.

Cancer research in 1992 was supported by $1.6 billion in direct funding at the National Cancer Institute alone.[176] Data from 1983 indicated that National Cancer Institute research funding constitutes approximately 50% of all cancer research funding from public and private sources.[177] A similar ratio in 1992 would mean that more than $3 billion were spent on cancer research nationally, which is more than thirty times the amount devoted to birth defects research. Yet, the total cost of cancer in the United States is approximately eight times that of birth defects, which is based on estimates from Rice et al.[178] This amount is conservative in terms of birth defect costs. In other words, relative to its estimated societal costs, cancer receives a far greater than proportionate share of research funding than does birth defects. This comparison does not mean that cancer research is overfunded relative to birth defects research. We do not know the potential benefit per additional research dollar spent in the two areas. Rather, our estimates of the societal costs of birth defects suggest that additional commitments of funds for prevention-oriented research may be a cost-effective strategy, one that could produce substantial savings in human and economic resources.

Endnotes to Chapter 7

1.Rice DP, Hodgson TA, Kopstein AN. The economic costs of illness: a replication and update. *Health Care Financing Review.* 1985;7(1).

2.Ibid.

3.Ibid.

4.Ibid.

5.Ibid.

6.Ibid.

7.Ibid.

8.Ibid.

9.National Foundation for Brain Research. *The Cost of Disorders of the Brain.* Washington, DC: Author; 1992.

10.Rice DP, et al. Ibid.

11.Ibid.

12.Lipscomb J. *Human Capital, Willingness-To-Pay and Cost-Effectiveness Analyses of Screening for Birth Defects in North Carolina.* Durham, North Carolina: Duke University; 1986.

13.Ibid.

14.Ibid.

15.Hu T, Sandifer FH. *Synthesis of Cost of Illness Methodology.* National Center for Health Services Research Contract No. 233-79-3010. Washington, DC: Public Services Laboratory, Georgetown University; 1981.

16.National Foundation for Brain Research. Ibid.

17.Romano PS, Waitzman NJ, Scheffler RM, Pi RD. Folic acid fortification of grain: an economic analysis. *Am J of Public Health.* 1995;85(5):667-677.

18.MRC Vitamin Study Research Group. Prevention of neural tube defects: results of the Medical Research Council vitamin study. *Lancet.* 1991;338:131-137.

19.Laurence KM, James N, Miller MH, Tennant GB, Campbell H. Double-blind randomized controlled trial of folate treatment before conception to prevent recurrence of neural-tube defects. *Br Med J.* 1981;282:1509-1511.

20.Czeizel AE, Dudas I. Prevention of the first occurrence of neural-tube defects by periconceptional vitamin supplementation. *N Engl J Med.* 1992;327:1832-1835.

21.Vergel RG, Sanchez LR, Heredero BL, Rodriguez PL, Martinez AJ. Primary prevention of neural tube defects with folic acid supplementation: Cuban experience. *Prenat Diagn.* 1990;10:149-152.

22.Milunsky A, Jick H, Jick SS, Bruell CL, MacLaughlin DS, Rothman KJ, Willett W. Multivitamin/folic acid supplementation in early pregnancy reduces the prevalence of neural tube defects. *JAMA.* 1989;262:2847-2852.

23.Centers for Disease Control. Recommendations for the use of folic acid to reduce the number of cases of spina bifida and other neural tube defects. *MMWR.* 1992;41(No. RR-14):1-7.

24.Food and Drug Administration, Food Advisory Committee, Subcommittee on Folic Acid. Transcript. Arlington, Virginia; November 23-24, 1992.

25.Grimes DA. Unplanned pregnancies in the United States. *Obstet Gynecol.* 1986;67:438-442.

26.Mills JL, Raymond E. Effects of recent research on recommendations for periconceptional folate supplement use. *Ann NY Acad Sci.* 1993;678:137-145.

27.Food standards: amendment of the standards of identity for enriched grain products to require addition of folic acid. *Federal Register.* October 14, 1993;58:53305-53312.

28.Romano PS, et al. Ibid.

29.Food and Drug Administration. Options document. Presented at the Folic Acid Subcommittee meeting. Crystal City, Virginia; April 15, 1993.

30.21 *Code of Federal Regulations* §137.

31.Putnam JJ, Allshouse JE. Food consumption, prices, and expenditures, 1970-90. *USDA Stat Bull.* 1992;840:1-20.

32.Hoffpauer DW. Rice enrichment for today. *Cereal Foods World.* 1992;37:757-759.

33.Food standards. Ibid.

34.Food standards. Ibid.

35.Walker ARP, Walker BF, Metz J. Acceptability trials of maize meal fortified with niacin, riboflavin, and folic acid. *S Afr Med J.* 1983;64:343-346.

36.Emodi AS, Scialpi L. Quality of bread fortification with ten micronutrients. *Cereal Chem.* 1980;57:1-3.

37.Kaunitz JD, Lindenbaum J. The bioavailability of folic acid added to wine. *Ann Intern Med.* 1977;87:542-545.

38.Holmes-Siedle M, Dennis J, Lindenbaum RH, Galliard A. Long-term effects of periconceptional multivitamin supplements for prevention of neural tube defects: a seven to 10 year follow up. *Arch Dis Child.* 1992;67:1436-1441.

39.Hellstrom L. Lack of toxicity of folic acid given in pharmacological doses to healthy volunteers. *Lancet.* 1971;i:59-61.

40.Smith DB, Racusen LC. Folate metabolism and the anticonvulsant efficacy of phenobarbital. *Arch Neurol.* 1973;28:18-22.

41.Hommes OR, Obbens EAMT. The epileptogenic action of Na-folate in the rat. *J Neurol Sci.* 1972;16:271-281.

42.Mauguiere F, Quoex C, Bello S. Epileptogenic properties of folic acid and N5 methyltetrahydrofolate in cat. *Epilepsia.* 1975;16:535-541.

43.Baylis EM, Crowley JM, Preece JM, Sylvester PE, Marks V. Influence of folic acid on blood-phenytoin levels. *Lancet.* 1971;i:62-64.

44.Jensen ON, Olesen OV. Subnormal serum folate due to anticonvulsive therapy: a double-blind study of the effect of folic acid treatment in patients with drug-induced subnormal serum folates. *Arch Neurol.* 1970;22:181-182.

45.Jensen ON, et al. Ibid.

46.Gibberd FB, Nicholls A, Wright MG. The influence of folic acid on the frequency of epileptic attacks. *Eur J Clin Pharmacol.* 1981;19:57-60.

47.Brown RS, Di Stanislao PT, Beaver WT, Bottomley WK. The administration of folic acid to institutionalized epileptic adults with phenytoin-induced gingival hyperplasia: a double-blind, randomized, placebo-controlled, parallel study. *Oral Surg Oral Med Oral Pathol.* 1991;71:565-568.

48.Backman N, Holm AK, Hanstrom L, Blomquist HK, Heijbel J, Safstrom G. Folate treatment of diphenylhydantoin-induced gingival hyperplasia. *Scan J Dent Res.* 1989;97:222-232.

49.Grant RHE, Stores OPR. Folic acid in folate-deficient patients with epilepsy. *Br Med J.* 1970;4:644-648.

50.Bowe JC, Cornish EJ, Dawson M. Evaluation of folic acid supplements in children taking phenytoin. *Dev Med Child Neurol.* 1971;13:343-354.

51.Mattson RH, Gallagher BB, Reynolds EH, Glass D. Folate therapy in epilepsy: a controlled study. *Arch Neurol.* 1973;29:78-81.

52.Norris JW, Pratt RF. A controlled study of folic acid in epilepsy. *Neurology.* 1971;21:659-664.

53.Houben PFM, Hommes OR, Knaven PJH. Anticonvulsant drugs and folic acid in young mentally retarded epileptic patients. *Epilesia.* 1971;12:235-247.

54.Ralston AJ, Snaith RP, Hinley JB. Effects of folic acid on fit-frequency and behaviour in epileptics on anticonvulsants. *Lancet.* 1970;i:867-868.

55.Morgan SL, Baggott JE, Vaughn WH, Young PK, Austin JV, Krumdieck CL, et al. The effect of folic acid supplementation on the toxicity of low-dose methotrexate in patients with rheumatoid arthritis. *Arthritis Rheum.* 1990;33:9-18.

56.Stewart KA, Mackenzie AH, Clough JD, Wilke WS. Folate supplementation in methotrexate-treated rheumatoid arthritis patients. *Sem Arthritis Rheum.* 1991;20:332-338.

57.Moore CV, Bierbaum OS, Welch AD, Wright LD. The activity of synthetic *Lactobacillus casei* factor (folic acid) as an anti-pernicious anemia substance. *J Lab Clin Med.* 1945;30:1056-1069.

58.Dudley GM III, Coltman CA. Resolution of ineffective erythropoiesis of pernicious anemia and "strongly suggestive" folate lack in response to folic acid. *Am J Clin Nutr.* 1970;23:147-155.

59.Sheehy TW, Rubini ME, Perez-Santiago E, Santini R Jr, Haddock J. Effect of "minute" and "titrated" amounts of folic acid on megaloblastic anemia of tropical sprue. *Blood.* 1961;18:623.

60.Herbert V. Diagnosis and treatment of folic acid deficiency. *Med Clin N Am.* 1962;46:1365.

61.Chosy JJ, Clatanoff DV, Schilling RF. Responses to small doses of folic acid in pernicious anemia. *Am J Clin Nutr.* 1962;10:349-350.

62.Herbert V. Current concepts in therapy: megaloblastic anemia. *New Engl J Med.* 1963;268:201-203.

63.Dudley GM III, Coltman CA. Ibid.

64.Hansen HA, Weinfeld A. Metabolic effects and diagnostic value of small doses of folic acid and B$_{12}$ in megaloblastic anemias. *Acta Med Scand.* 1962;172:427-443.

65.Marshall RA, Jandl JH. Response to physiologic doses of folic acid in the megaloblastic anemias. *Arch Intern Med.* 1960;105:352.

66.Schwartz SO, Kaplan SR, Armstrong BF. The long-term evaluation of folic acid in the treatment of pernicious anemia. *J Lab Clin Med.* 1950;35:894-898.

67.Schwartz SO, et al. Ibid.

68.Heinle RW, Welch AD. Folic acid in pernicious anemia: failure to prevent neurologic relapse. *JAMA.* 1947;133:739-741.

69.Hall BE, Watkins CH. Experience with pteroylglutamic acid in treatment of pernicious anemia. *J Lab Clin Med.* 1947;32:622-634.

70.Baldwin JN, Dalessio DJ. Folic acid therapy and spinal-cord degeneration in pernicious anemia. *New Engl J Med.* 1961;264:1339-1342.

71.Will JJ, Mueller JF, Brodine C, Kiely CE, Friedman B, Hawkins VR, et al. Folic acid and vitamin B$_{12}$ in pernicious anemia: studies on patients treated with these substances over a ten-year period. *J Lab Clin Med.* 1959;53:22-38.

72.Meyer LM. Folic acid in the treatment of pernicious anemia. *Blood.* 1947;2:50-62.

73.Allen RH, Stabler SP, Savage DG, Lindenbaum J. Diagnosis of cobalamin deficiency I: usefulness of serum methylmalonic acid and total homocysteine concentrations. *Am J Hematol.* 1990;34:90-98.

74.Vilter RW, Horrigan D, Mueller JF, Jarrold T, Vilter CF, Hawkins V, et al. Studies on the relationships of vitamin B_{12}, folic acid, thymine, uracil, and methyl group donors in persons with pernicious anemia and related megaloblastic anemias. *Blood.* 1950;5:695-717.

75.Ross JF, Belding H, Paegel BL. The development and progression of subacute combined degeneration of the spinal cord in patients with pernicious anemia treated with synthetic pteroylglutamic (folic) acid. *Blood.* 1948;3:68-90.

76.Bethell FH, Sturgis CC. The relation of therapy in pernicious anemia to changes in the nervous system: early and late results in a series of cases observed for periods of not less than ten years, and early results of treatment with folic acid. *Blood.* 1948;3:57-67.

77.Victor M, Lear AA. Subacute combined degeneration of the spinal cord. Current concepts of the disease process: value of serum vitamin B_{12} determinations in clarifying some of the common clinical problems. *Am J Med.* 1956;20:896-911.

78.Israels MCG, Wilkinson JF. Risk of neurological complications in pernicious anemia treated with folic acid. *Br Med J.* 1949;2:1072-1075.

79.Ellison ABC. Pernicious anemia masked by multivitamins containing folic acid. *JAMA.* 1960;173:240-243.

80.Pedersen AB, Mosbech J. Morbidity of pernicious anemia: Incidence, prevalence, and treatment in a Danish county. *Acta Med Scand.* 1969;185:449-452.

81.Borch K, Lindberg G. Prevalence and incidence of pernicious anemia: an evaluation for gastric screening. *Scand J Gastroenterol,* 1984;19:154-160.

82.Israels MCG, Wilkinson JF. Ibid.

83.Graves EJ. Detailed diagnoses and procedures, National Hospital Discharge Survey, 1989. *Vital Health Stat.* 1991;13(108).

84.Lewin-ICF. *The cost of disorders of the brain.* Washington, DC: National Foundation for Brain Research; 1992.

85.Lewin-ICF. Ibid.

86.Hodgson TA, Kopstein AN. Health care expenditures for major diseases in 1980. *Health Care Financ Rev.* 1984;5:1-12.

87.Rice DP, Hodgson TA, Kopstein AN. The economic costs of illness: a replication and update. *Health Care Financ Rev.* 1985;7:61-80.

88.Healton EB, Savage DG, Brust JCM, Garrett TJ, Lindenbaum J. Neurologic aspects of cobalamin deficiency. *Medicine.* 1991;70:229-245.

89.MRC Vitamin Study Research Group. Ibid.

90.Lawrence KM, et al. Ibid.

91.Smithells RW, Sheppard S, Schorah CJ, Seller MJ, Nevin NC, Harris R, et al. Possible prevention of neural-tube defects by periconceptional vitamin supplementation. *Lancet.* 1980;1:339-340.

92.Smithells RW, Sheppard S, Schorah CJ, et al. Apparent prevention of neural tube defects by periconceptional multivitamin supplementation. *Arch Dis Child.* 1981;56:911-918.

93.Smithells RW, Seller MJ, Harris R, Fielding DW, Schorah CJ, Nevin NC, et al. Further experience of vitamin supplementation for prevention of neural tube defect recurrences. *Lancet.* 1983;1:1027-1031.

94.Smithells RW, Sheppard S, Wald J, Schorah CJ. Prevention of neural tube defect recurrences in Yorkshire: final report. *Lancet.* 1989;2:498-499.

95.Czeizel AE, Dudas I. Ibid.

96.Vergel RG, et al. Ibid.

97.Mulinare J, Cordero JF, Erickson JD, Berry RJ. Periconceptional use of multivitamins and the occurrence of neural tube defects. *JAMA.* 1988; 260:3141-3145.

98.Werler MM, Shapiro S, Mitchell AA. Periconceptional folic acid exposure and risk of occurrent neural tube defects. *JAMA.* 1993;269:1257-1261.

99.Mills JL, Rhoads GG, Simpson JL, Cunningham GC, Conley MR, Lassman MR, et al. The absence of a relation between the periconceptional use of vitamins and neural tube defects. *New Engl J Med.* 1989;321:430-435.

100.Bower C, Stanley FJ. Dietary folate as a risk factor for neural-tube defects: evidence from a case-control study in Western Australia. *Med J Aust.* 1989;150:613-619.

101.Winship KA, Cahal DA, Weber JCP, Griffin JP. Maternal drug histories and central nervous system anomalies. *Arch Dis Child.* 1984;59:1052-1060.

102.Bower C, Stanley FJ. Periconceptional vitamin supplementation and neural tube defects; evidence from a case-control study in Western Australia and a review of recent publications. *J Epidemiol Community Health.* 1992;46:157-161.

103.Watson Duff EM, Cooper ES. Neural tube defects in Jamaica following Hurricane Gilbert. *Am J Public Health.* 1994;84:473-476.

104.Milunsky A, et al. Ibid.

105.Mills JL, et al. Ibid.

106.Colman N, Green R, Metz J. Prevention of folate deficiency by food fortification. II. Absorption of folic acid from fortified staple foods. *Am J Clin Nutr.* 1975;28:459-464.

107.Colman N, Larsen JV, Barker M, Barker EA, Green R, Metz J. Prevention of folate deficiency by food fortification. III. effect in pregnant subjects of varying amounts of added folic acid. *Am J Clin Nutr.* 1975;28:465-470.

108.Milunsky A, et al. Ibid.

109.Werler MM, et al. Ibid.

110.Bower C, et al. Ibid.

111.Yates JRW, Ferguson-Smith MA, Senkin A, Guzman-Rodrigues R, White M, Clarke BJ. Is disordered folate metabolism the basis for the genetic predisposition to neural tube defects? *Clin Genet.* 1987;31:279-287.

112.Milunsky A, et al. Ibid.

113.Ibid.

114.Ibid.

115.Werler MM, et al. Ibid.

116.Bower C, et al. Ibid.

117.Bailey LB. Evaluation of a new recommended dietary allowance for folate. *J Am Diet Assoc.* 1992;92:463-468.

118.McPartlin J, Halligan A, Scott JM, Darling M, Weir DG. Accelerated folate breakdown in pregnancy. *Lancet.* 1993;341:148-149.

119.Sauberlich HE, Kretsch MJ, Skala JH, Johnson HL, Taylor PC. Folate requirement and metabolism in nonpregnant women. *Am J Clin Nutr.* 1987;46:1016-1028.

120.Hawkes JG, Villota R. Folates in foods: Reactivity, stability during processing, and nutritional implications. *Crit Rev Food Sci Nutr.* 1989;28:439-538.

121.Thenen SW. Folacin content of supplemental foods for pregnancy. *J Am Diet Assoc.* 1982;80:237-241.

122.Subar AF, Block G, James LD. Folate intake and food sources in the US population. *Am J Clin Nutr.* 1989;50:508-516.

123.Block G, Abrams B. Vitamin and mineral status of women of childbearing potential. *Ann NY Acad Sci.* 1993;678:244-254.

124.Alaimo K, McDowell MA, Briefel RR, et al. Dietary intake of vitamins, minerals, and fiber of persons ages 2 months and over in the United States: third National Health and Nutrition Examination Survey, Phase 1, 1988-91. Advance data from vital and health statistics; no. 258. Hyattsville, Maryland: National Center for Health Statistics; 1994.

125.Moss AJ, Levy AS, Kim I, Park YK. Use of vitamin and mineral supplements in the United States: current users, types of products, and nutrients. Advance data from vital and health statistics; no. 174. Hyattsville, Maryland: National Center for Health Statistics; 1989.

126.Mills JL, et al. Ibid.

127.Werler MM, et al. Ibid.

128.Mulinare J, et al. Ibid.

129.Mills JL, et al. Ibid.

130.Werler MM, et al. Ibid.

131.Food and Drug Administration. Ibid.

132.Food standards. Ibid.

133.Mertz W, Tsui JC, Judd JT, Reiser S, Hallfrisch J, Morris ER, Steele PD, Lashley E. What are people really eating? The relation between energy intake derived from estimated diet records and intake determined to maintain body weight. *Am J Clin Nutr.* 1991;54:291-295.

134.Waitzman NJ, Romano PS, Scheffler RM. Estimates of the economic costs of birth defects. *Inquiry.* 1994;31:188-205.

135.Iyengar L, Rajalakshmi K. Effect of folic acid supplement on birth weights of infants. *Am J Obstet Gynecol.* 1975;122:332-336.

136.Baumslag N, Edelstein J, Metz J. Reduction of incidence of prematurity by folic acid supplementation in pregnancy. *Br Med J.* 1970;1:16-17.

137.Larroque B, Kaminski M, Lelong N, d' Herbomez M, Dehaene P, Querleu D, et al. Folate status during pregnancy: relationship with alcohol consumption, other maternal risk factors and pregnancy outcome. *Eur J Obstet Gynecol Repro Biol.* 1992;43:19-27.

138.Mukherjee MD, Sandstead HH, Ratnaparkhi MV, Johnson LK, Milne DB, Stelling HP. Maternal zinc, iron, folic acid, and protein nutriture and outcome of human pregnancy. *Am J Clin Nutr.* 1984;40:496-507.

139.Fletcher J, Gurr A, Fellingham FR, Prankerd TAJ, Brant HA, Menzies DN. The value of folic acid supplements in pregnancy. *J Obstet Gynaecol Br Commonw.* 1971;78:781-785.

140.Rolschau J, Date J, Kristoffersen K. Folic acid supplement and intrauterine growth. *Acta Obstet Gynecol Scand.* 1979;58:343-346.

141.Giles PF, Harcourt AG, Whiteside MG. The effect of prescribing folic acid during pregnancy on birth-weight and duration of pregnancy: a double-blind trial. *Med J Aust.* 1971;2:17-21.

142.Blot I, Papiernik E, Kaltwasser JP, Werner E, Tchernia G. Influence of routine administration of folic acid and iron during pregnancy. *Gynecol Obstet Invest.* 1981;12:294-304.

143.Tolorova M. Periconceptional supplement with vitamins and folic acid to prevent recurrence of cleft lip. *Lancet.* 1982;2:217.

144.Conway H. Effect of supplemental vitamin therapy on the limitation of incidence of cleft lip and cleft palate in humans. *Plast Reconstr Surg.* 1958;22:450-453.

145.Briggs RM. Vitamin supplementation as a possible factor in the incidence of cleft lip/palate deformities in humans. *Clin Plast Surg.* 1976;3:647-652.

146.Czeizel AE, Dudas I. Ibid.

147.Bower C, Stanley FJ. Dietary folate and nonneural midline birth defects: no evidence of an association from a case-control study in western Australia. *Am J Med Genet.* 1992;44:647-650.

148.Eto I, Krumdieck CL. Role of vitamin B_{12} and folate deficiencies and carcinogenesis. *Adv Exp Med Biol.* 1986;206:313-330.

149.Butterworth CE Jr, Hatch KD, Gore H, Mueller H, Krumdieck CL. Improvement in cervical dysplasia associated with folic acid therapy in users of oral contraceptives. *Am J Clin Nutr.* 1982;35:73-82.

150.Butterworth CE Jr, Hatch KD, Soong SJ, Cole P, Tamura T, Sauberlich HE, et al. Oral folic acid supplementation for cervical dysplasia: a clinical intervention trial. *Am J Obstet Gynecol.* 1992;166:803-809.

151.Potischman N, Brinton LA, Laiming VA, Reeves WC, Brenes MM, Herrero R, et al. A case-control study of serum folate levels and invasive cervical cancer. *Cancer Res.* 1991;51:4785-4789.

152.Ziegler RG, Brinton LA, Hammon RF, Lehman HF, Levine RS, et al. Diet and the risk of invasive cervical cancer among white women in the United States. *Am J Epidemiol.* 1990;132:432-445.

153.Verreault R, Chu J, Mandelson M, Shy K. A case-control study of diet and invasive cervical cancer. *Int J Cancer.* 1989;43:1050-1054.

154.Lashner BA, Heidenreich PA, Su GL, Kane SV, Hanauer SB. Effect of folate supplementation on the incidence of dysplasia and cancer in chronic ulcerative colitis: A case-control study. *Gastroenterology.* 1989;97:255-259.

155.Heimburger DC, Alexander CB, Birch R, Butterworth CE Jr, Bailey WC, Krumdieck CL. Improvement in bronchial squamous metaplasia in smokers treated with folate and vitamin B_{12}: report of a preliminary randomized double-blind intervention trial. *JAMA.* 1988;259:1525-1530.

156.Selhub J, Jacques PF, Wilson PWF, Rush D, Rosenberg IH. Vitamin status and intake as primary determinants of homocysteinemia in an elderly population. *JAMA.* 1993;270:2693-2698.

157.Stampfer MJ, Malinow MR, Willett WC, et al. A prospective study of plasma homocyst(e)ine and risk of myocardial infarction in US physicians. *JAMA.* 1992;268:877-881.

158.Brattstrom LE, Israelsson B, Jeppsson JO, Hultberg BL. Folic acid: an innocuous means to reduce plasma homocyst(e)ine. *Scand J Clin Lab Invest.* 1988;48:215-221.

159.Centers for Disease Control. Spina bifida incidence at birth: United States, 1983-1990. *MMWR.* 41(27):497-500.

160.National Center for Health Statistics. Births, marriages, divorces, and deaths for 1992. *Monthly Vital Stat Rep.* 1993;41(12):1-24.

161.Worley G, Rosenfeld LR, Lipscomb J. Financial counseling for families of children with chronic disabilities. *Dev Med Child Neurol.* 1991;33:679-689.

162.Salkever DS. Parental opportunity costs and other economic costs of children's disabling conditions. In: Hobbs N, Perrin JM, eds. *Issues in the care of children with chronic illness.* San Francisco, California: Jossey-Bass; 1985:864-878.

163.Evans O, Tew B, Payne H, Laurence KM. Medical and social service provision for families of children with NTD. *Z Kinderchir.* 1987;42(suppl I):17-20.

164.Evans O, Tew B, Laurence KM. The fathers of children with spina bifida. *Z Kinderchir.* 1986;41(suppl I):42-44.

165.Carr J, Pearson A, Halliwell M. The effect of disability on family life. *Z Kinderchir.* 1983;38(suppl II):103-106.

166.Walker JH, Thomas M, Russell IT. Spina bifida-and the parents. *Develop Med Child Neurol.* 1971;13:462-476.

167.Tew BJ, Laurence KM, Payne H, Rawnsley K. Marital stability following the birth of a child with spina bifida. *Brit J Psychiatr.* 1977;131:79-82.

168.Martin P. Marital breakdown in families of patients with spina bifida cystica. *Develop Med Child Neurol.* 1975;17:757-764.

169.Harrison MR, Adzick NS, Longaker MT, Goldberg JD, Rosen MA, Filly RA, et al. Successful repair in utero of a fetal diaphragmatic hernia after removal of herniated viscera from the left thorax. *New Engl J Med.* 1990;322:1582-1584.

170.Longaker MT, Golbus MS, Filly RA, Rosen MA, Chang SW, Harrison MR. Maternal outcome after open fetal surgery: a review of the first 17 human cases. *JAMA.* 1991;265:737-741.

171.Harrison MR, Adzick NS. The fetus as patient: surgical considerations. *Ann Surg.* 1991;213:279-291.

172.Chavez GF, Mulinare J, Cordero JF. Maternal cocaine use during early pregnancy as a risk factor for congenital urogenital anomalies. *JAMA.* 1989;262:795-798.

173.Cousins L. Etiology and prevention of congenital anomalies among infants of overt diabetic women. *Clin Obstet Gynecol.* 1991;34:481-493.

174.Scheffler RM, Feuchtbaum LB, Phibbs CS. Prevention: the cost-effectiveness of the California Diabetes and Pregnancy Program. *Am J Public Health.* 1992;82:168-175.

175.Figures for the March of Dimes were from the March of Dimes Annual Report in 1991.

176.U.S. Department of Health and Human Services, Public Health Service, National Institutes of Health. *Factbook: National Cancer Institute, 1992.* Washington, DC: Author; 1992.

177.US Department of Health and Human Services, Public Health Service, National Institutes of Health. *NCI Factbook: National Cancer Program, 1983.* Washington, DC: Author; 1983.

178.Rice DP, et al. Ibid.

Appendix 1

Description of Birth Defects

This appendix provides a detailed description of each of the birth defects for which an estimate was made of cost.

Spina Bifida

Spina bifida develops during pregnancy when the neural tube fails to close properly as the embryo is developing. Characteristically, the spinal arches do not fuse and a fluid-filled sac protrudes from the infant's back. In 90% of cases, this sac includes an abnormal spinal cord and surrounding membranes and is, therefore, called a *myelomeningocele*. Myelomeningoceles cause neurologic defects that relate to the level of spine affected by the malformation. For example, sacral malformations cause bowel, bladder, and sexual dysfunction. At the lumbar level, spina bifida also causes paralysis of the legs. This paralysis may be partial or total, depending whether the lesion is low or high in the lumbar spine. In addition to these impairments, cervical spina bifida also causes paralysis of the arms. Among live-born infants, approximately 21% of myelomeningoceles are sacral, 42% are lumbosacral, 27% are thoracolumbar, and 10% are thoracic or cervical.

Most infants with spina bifida also have the Arnold-Chiari malformation, a disorder in which the flow of cerebrospinal fluid, the fluid that bathes the brain and spinal cord, is blocked because the base of the brain is displaced downward into the spinal canal. When this disorder is left untreated, hydrocephalus develops as cerebrospinal fluid accumulates in and around the brain, causing compression of the brain within the rigid confines of the skull.

Although the cause of spina bifida has not been established, children of diabetic mothers, mothers who take sulfonamides or antihistamines during pregnancy,[1] folate-deficient mothers,[2,3,4,5] and mothers with prior affected children[6] are at especially high risk. Widespread screening of pregnant women and improved nutrition may explain[7] the significant decreases in the birth prevalence of spina bifida noted in Europe[8,9] and the United States.[10]

Children and adults with spina bifida have a variety of associated health problems. Relatively few (6%) have malformations outside the central nervous system, but such defects can include cleft lip or palate, constriction or closure (atresia) of the esophagus, diaphragmatic hernia, and kidney anomalies.[11] Several of these anomalies are described later in this appendix. Atrophy of the optic nerve and an inability to focus both eyes on the same object (strabismus) have been reported to occur in 17% and 42% of patients, respectively.[12] Between 20% and 30% of children with spina bifida develop epilepsy, which usually can be controlled with anticonvulsants.[13,14,15] Congenital curvature of the spine (scoliosis) occurs in approximately 15% of cases.[16] Poor neuromuscular control leads to a moderate-to-severe acquired curvature in nearly all children with thoracic or high-lumbar lesions[17] and a mild-to-moderate curvature in 70% to 80% of infants with low-lumbar or sacral lesions. Dysfunction of the arms, presumably related to hydrocephalus, has been noted in approximately 45% of patients (even those with lumbar or sacral lesions).[18,19] Approximately 30% to 50% of children with spina bifida become significantly overweight,[20] which may lead to obstruction of the airway during sleep and eventually to heart failure. Pressure sores and other skin problems affect approximately 70% of adolescents and young adults with spina bifida.[21,22] Bladder dysfunction is almost always present, although 87% of children over five years of age achieve urinary continence.[23]

The treatment of spina bifida may begin before birth because infants diagnosed with the disorder during pregnancy are often delivered by cesarean section to preserve their motor function.[24] During 1988, the index year for our study, however, vaginal delivery was still considered acceptable in such cases.[25]

The spinal defect is surgically closed within a few days after birth to minimize the risks of bacterial contamination[26] and neurologic deterioration. Even though some clinicians favor the selective treatment of infants who are "considered likely to benefit,"[27,28,29] legal and ethical concerns have led medical centers in the United States to use aggressive measures in treating nearly all infants with spina bifida.[30] Tethered-cord syndrome, which produces back pain or decreased motor or bladder function, occurs in 10% to 20% of patients within several years after closure;[31,32,33] it usually responds to surgical intervention. In order to prevent or treat hydrocephalus, more than 90% of infants with spina bifida receive a ventriculoperitoneal shunt that carries fluid from the head to the abdominal cavity where it is safely resorbed. As many as 10% of these shunts later become infected. In patients with severe scoliosis, surgery to fuse vertebrae and stabilize the spine may be necessary.[34] Patients who were treated with urinary diversion procedures in the 1960s and 1970s have a high risk of chronic kidney disease, with resulting hypertension,[35] because of abnormal reflux of urine back to the kidneys.[36,37] This complication should become less prevalent[38] as more patients are regularly catheterizing themselves to drain their urine.[39] Patients with spina bifida whose kidneys fail are candidates for hemodialysis or transplantation.[40]

Even with treatment, children with spina bifida do not live a normal life span. In addition, there are significant problems related to their social isolation.[41] Although at least 50% of affected adolescents and young adults participate in nonathletic activities with friends, most have difficulty with heterosexual relationships.[42,43,44,45] Cross-sectional studies of adults with spina bifida show that 20% to 40% are competitively employed, and up to 19% work in sheltered workshops.[46,47,48,49]

Conotruncal Heart Anomalies: Truncus Arteriosus

In normal infants, oxygen-saturated (red) blood is pumped out of the heart' s left side, through the major arteries, and then throughout the body via the systemic circulation. Some of this oxygen-saturated blood feeds the heart muscle itself via the coronary circulation. After nourishing the body with oxygen, desaturated (blue) blood is carried through the major veins to the heart's right side, which sends it via the pulmonary circulation to the lungs, where it is again saturated with oxygen and then returned to the left side of the heart.

In infants with truncus arteriosus, a single arterial trunk supplies mixed saturated and desaturated blood to the pulmonary, systemic, and coronary circulations. An abnormal valve in this arterial trunk overrides a defect in the muscular wall (ventricular septum) that separates the left and right ventricles, which are the two pumping chambers of the heart. Constriction (stenosis) or backflow (regurgitation) of blood across this valve occurs in 10% to 15% of patients.[50] The cause of conotruncal anomalies, including truncus arteriosus, is unknown.

Heart defects associated with this condition include underdevelopment of the aortic arch, displacement or stenosis at the origin of the coronary arteries, and absence of the main pulmonary artery supplying the lungs.[51] Affected children suffer primarily from congestive heart failure, resulting from abnormal shunting of saturated blood through the truncus into the pulmonary circulation. Constriction of the pulmonary arteries rarely restricts blood flow to the lungs and causes cyanosis, a condition in which the child's skin and mucous membranes appear dark blue because of insufficient oxygen in the blood. The long-term prognosis for infants who do not undergo surgery is dismal; that is, approximately 75% die from heart failure before their first birthday, and most survivors have severe pulmonary vascular disease. Surgery to palliate the condition such as banding the pulmonary artery to reduce blood flow to the lungs does not substantially improve long-term survival.[52]

Corrective surgery for this condition is performed when the infant is six to twelve weeks of age. During surgery, the pulmonary arteries are separated from the common arterial trunk, and the defect in the ventricular septum is closed. A valve-containing conduit is constructed from natural aortic tissue or Dacron; this conduit is placed to connect the right ventricle with the pulmonary arteries. The truncal valve requires replacement in as many as 6% of patients;[53,54] a smaller percentage have narrowed valves that can be opened surgically. Of 106 infants younger than six months of age who were treated at one medical center, 6% died before surgery and 10% died during or shortly after surgery.[55] Three other infants (3%) died later. Results were similar in another study.[56] Survival analyses indicate that between 15% and 50% of these conduits fail and require replacement within five years.[57,58,59] Even if they do not fail, routine replacement is recommended when the child is twelve years old because of the child's growth. Children may experience complications as a result of these periodic conduit dilations or replacements.

Conotruncal Heart Anomalies: Transposition of the Great Arteries

In newborn infants, the most common cardiac cause of cyanosis is a complete transposition of the great arteries. In this condition, the aorta arises from the right ventricle and the pulmonary artery arises from the left ventricle of the heart. As a result, desaturated (blue) blood returning from the body is ejected into the aorta, and oxygen-saturated (red) blood returning from the lungs is sent back to the lungs through the pulmonary artery. The only routes by which desaturated blood can get to the lungs are through a defect in the ventricular septum, which is a persistent connection between the aorta and the main pulmonary artery (patent ductus arteriosus), or a persistent opening between the left and right atria (patent foramen ovale). The last two of these connections are present in all fetuses, but they normally close off shortly after birth.

Associated cardiac defects include obstruction of the outflow of blood from the left or right ventricle. Children with transposition have reduced severely levels of oxygen in the blood and impaired tissue metabolism. In the 20% of children who have an associated ventricular septal defect,[60] excessive blood flow to the lungs often results in congestive heart failure and pulmonary vascular disease. Without surgery, transposition is almost invariably fatal. Early treatment to palliate the condition may include intravenous medications that help keep the ductus arteriosus open and insertion of a balloon into the ventricular septum that enlarges the interatrial communication and allows more saturated blood to enter the systemic circulation.[61] Despite these measures, approximately 10% of infants succumb to oxygen deprivation or heart failure during the first thirty days of life without surgery.[62,63]

Two surgical approaches have been devised to correct transposition: (a) the arterial switch and (b) the atrial switch. During an arterial switch, the aorta and main pulmonary artery are cut above the aortic and pulmonary valves, the vessels are switched, and the coronary arteries are transplanted to the pulmonary artery in order to receive saturated blood pumped out of the left ventricle. This operation must be performed during the first few weeks of life before the left ventricle regresses in response to the lower pressure in the pulmonary circulation (which occurs naturally after birth).[64] Among 302 infants with simple transposition who underwent an arterial switch, 86% were still alive at one month, 84% were alive at one year, and survival remained stable thereafter. Among sixty-eight infants with transposition and large ventricular septal defects, survival was 78% at one month and at one year. A study from the Netherlands yielded similar findings.[65] Approximately 10% of patients require another operation within one year, often because of obstruction of the new pulmonary artery or a residual septal defect. Over longer periods of follow-up, fewer than 5% of patients have impaired functional status or diminished cardiac function. However, scarring at the origin of the transplanted coronary arteries may lead to angina and other signs of cardiac ischemia.[66]

During an atrial switch, the atrial septum is replaced with a flap of tissue (often derived from the outer lining of the heart) that diverts desaturated blood from the right atrium to the left ventricle and diverts oxygen-saturated blood from the left atrium to the right ventricle. In this surgery, the left ventricle retains its abnormal connection to the pulmonary artery, and the right ventricle retains its abnormal connection to the aorta. Even though the percentage of infants surviving after an atrial switch is comparable to that after arterial switch,[67] arrhythmias develop in 30% to 80% within ten years[68,69,70,71] despite efforts to protect the heart's intrinsic pacemaker.[72] Between 3% and 10% of children with this disorder eventually require an artificial pacemaker.[73,74] Leakage across the diverting tissue flap is a common, but less serious, complication. Because the right ventricle is forced to pump against high pressures, the heart's response to exercise is often abnormal, and cardiac dysfunction may occur in 10% of children within ten years. Arrhythmias and heart failure lead to death in approximately 11% of patients between thirty days and ten years after surgery.[75]

Conotruncal Heart Anomalies: Double-Outlet Right Ventricle

Double-outlet right ventricle (DORV) is a heterogeneous category of rare malformations in which the aorta and the pulmonary artery originate from the right ventricle, and a ventricular septal defect provides the only outlet from the left ventricle. The Taussig-Bing malformation is a form of DORV that resembles a transposition in which the pulmonary artery overrides the ventricular septal defect.[76] Associated heart defects may include complex lesions of the atrial or ventricular septum, patent ductus arteriosus, dextrocardia (in which the heart is located on the right side of the chest), and narrowing (stenosis) or regurgitation (backflow) of the atrioventricular valves.[77] The clinical manifestations of these defects vary. Children with associated stenosis of the pulmonary valve become blue (cyanotic) and tolerate exercise poorly, whereas children without such stenosis develop heart failure and pulmonary vascular disease. Without surgery, the long-term prognosis is poor.

Palliative procedures such as banding the pulmonary artery or creating a shunt to alter blood flow to the lungs are performed shortly after birth, when necessary. Definitive repair, which is done when the child is six to twenty-four months old, usually involves placing a prosthetic patch to direct blood from the left ventricle to the aorta. This procedure also may involve enlarging the ventricular septal defect, correcting any associated atrial septal defect, and reconstructing the right ventricle's outflow pathway. The Taussig-Bing malformation must be corrected by atrial or arterial switch, although the arterial switch is preferred. Death occurs soon after DORV repair in 15% of infants or fewer and usually results from poor cardiac output or hemorrhage.[78] Approximately 25% of children who survive surgery die later in childhood. Most of those deaths are probably related to arrhythmias.[79]

Contruncal Heart Anomalies: Single Ventricle

In single-ventricle hearts, there is only one functional ventricle (pumping chamber) in which oxygen-saturated blood returning from the lungs mixes with desaturated blood from the rest of the body.

Associated cardiac anomalies may include malpositioning of the great arteries, stenosis at the pulmonic valve or just below the aortic valve, defects of the atrial septum, abnormal return of blood from the lungs, and severe narrowing (coarctation) of the aorta. Associated anomalies not involving the heart such as scoliosis and the absence of a spleen are found in 20% to 40% of infants.[80,81] Affected children tolerate exercise poorly and become blue, with a resulting increase in the concentration of red blood cells. Unless the infant has an associated narrowing of the pulmonary vessels, excessive blood flow to the lungs results in heart failure and pulmonary vascular disease. Without surgery, at least 70% of affected children die before they are sixteen years old.

The most common type of corrective surgery is the Fontan procedure in which desaturated blood is directed from the right atrium of the heart through a conduit or opening to the pulmonary arteries. At many medical centers, this operation is performed in two stages: (a) The pulmonary arteries are disconnected from the single ventricle during early infancy, and (b) the conduit is constructed when the child is eighteen to thirty-six months of age. Among 156 infants treated at one center,[82] survival was 82% at one year, 73% at four years, and 57% at ten years;[83] two other medical centers have reported 75% short-term survival[84] and 71% survival at ten years.[85] Within ten years after Fontan surgery, 14% of children must have another operation to clear obstruction of the conduit.[86] Replacement of the original conduit with a larger conduit is also sometimes necessary.[87] Among seventy-seven infants surveyed six months to seven years after undergoing Fontan surgery, 10% had markedly limited activity but only 3% were unable to work or attend school.[88]

A less common but promising procedure involves dividing the single ventricle into two chambers (septation) with a Dacron or Teflon patch. Although septation creates a better physiologic state than the Fontan procedure, it is best performed in patients who do not have significant pulmonic stenosis or enlargement of the heart chambers.[89] In the past, 36% to 47% of infants who underwent septation died before leaving the hospital, but better outcomes recently have been reported in a series of carefully selected patients.

Conotruncal Heart Anomalies: Tetralogy of Fallot

Tetralogy of Fallot is characterized by obstruction of outflow from the right ventricle, a large defect in the ventricular septum, an unusually positioned aorta overriding the septal defect, and increased thickness of the right ventricular wall.[90] Associated cardiac anomalies may include pulmonic stenosis, underdevelopment of the pulmonary arteries, an atrial septal defect, a right-sided aortic arch, and anomalies of the coronary arteries. Children with this defect seldom have anomalies unrelated to the heart. Because obstruction of outflow from the right ventricle causes desaturated blood to be shunted across the ventricular septal defect to the systemic circulation, children with this defect become cyanotic (blue). Fluctuations in vascular resistance cause transient episodes of increased shunting of blood, which is manifested by shortness of breath and decreased blood oxygen levels. If tetralogy is untreated, these spells become frequent and unresponsive to medical therapy.

Children with tetralogy usually undergo surgical correction when they are three to twelve months of age, although some surgeons wait longer if the child has no symptoms. Definitive repair includes closure of the ventricular septal defect with a patch, removal of the outflow obstruction from the right ventricle, and dilation or surgical division (commissurotomy) of the pulmonic valve, if necessary. Newborn infants with poorly developed pulmonary arteries may require placement of a shunt soon after birth in order to augment blood flow to their lungs. After definitive repair, 3% to 8% of infants die before leaving the hospital.[91,92] Approximately 87% to 90% of treated children are alive ten years after the procedure, and 85% are still alive after twenty-five to twenty-six years.[93,94,95,96] From 5% to 15% of children require a second operation within thirteen years. Most surviving children have excellent functional status.[97]

Cleft Lip or Palate

Cleft lip with or without cleft palate is the most common craniofacial malformation. Approximately 50% of affected children have clefts of both the lip and the palate; the remaining have only cleft lip (25%) or cleft palate (25%).[98] Cleft palate may involve only the soft palate, both the soft and hard palates, or the entire roof of the mouth. Wide clefts may be associated with defects of the nasal septum and with an open communication between the nose and mouth. Submucous clefts are limited to the palatal muscles; the overlying mucous membranes are intact. Cleft lip may be in the midline, or it may affect one or both sides of the face. A great variety of factors is involved in the development of cleft deformities, but genetics and certain teratogens such as alcohol have been implicated.

More than 50% of patients with isolated cleft palates have other anomalies[99,100,101,102] such as underdevelopment of the facial bones, an abnormally wide distance between the eyes, an abnormally small head (microcephaly), conotruncal heart defects,[103] defects of the abdominal wall, and dental malformations. Among patients with cleft lip (with or without cleft palate), associated anomalies occur in only 14% to 35%.[104] Children with cleft deformities may suck ineffectively and may suffer from swallowing problems and chronic aspiration of food into the lungs. These children also may be delayed in learning to talk or may have distorted speech.[105] Other problems associated with cleft deformities include crossbite,[106] recurrent middle ear and sinus infections, reading disabilities,[107] and inadequate social relationships.[108,109]

Currently, the management of cleft deformities includes surgical closure of cleft lip during the first months of life, initial repair of the palate at six to eighteen months of age, closure of residual defects with bone grafts during adolescence, and orthodontic and speech therapy as needed. Long-term outcomes generally are excellent, although associated anomalies may shorten the child's survival.

Tracheoesophageal Fistula

Tracheoesophageal fistula and/or esophageal atresia are the most common congenital anomalies of the esophagus. An atretic esophagus ends in a blind pouch with no connection to the stomach. Five types of anomalies have been described: (a) esophageal atresia with an abnormal channel (fistula) connecting the lower esophageal segment and the trachea (85% to 88% of cases[110,111]), (b) esophageal atresia without a fistula (7% to 8%), (c) esophageal atresia with a fistula between the upper esophageal segment and the trachea (0% to 1%), (d) esophageal atresia with separate fistulas connecting both segments to the trachea (1% to 2%), and (e) tracheoesophageal fistula without esophageal atresia (2% to 3%). The causes or mechanisms of these esophageal defects are unknown.

Esophageal atresia typically is evident on the first day of life, as the infant drools, regurgitates milk, coughs, chokes, or becomes cyanotic.[112] Children later develop abdominal distention as inhaled air passes from the trachea to the stomach; in turn, stomach acid refluxes into the lungs. Tracheoesophageal fistula without esophageal atresia often manifests later in childhood with chronic cough, recurrent pneumonia, hyperreactive airways, and failure to thrive. Approximately 30% to 55% of patients have associated anomalies such as a patent ductus arteriosus, defects of the atrial or ventricular septum, tetralogy of Fallot, anomalies of the anus or rectum, atresia of the small intestine, and defects of the spinal column.[113,114,115]

When a full-term infant with esophageal atresia lacks other severe anomalies, surgical correction is undertaken within several days after birth. The preferred approach is primary anastomosis or surgical attachment of the segments of esophagus above and below the site of atresia. Long gaps are bridged by progressively stretching the upper segment or by using a piece of stomach or colon. Mortality after surgery depends on the infant's Waterston classification: Group A has a birthweight greater than 2,500 g and no associated anomalies—or only minor ones; group B has a birthweight of 1,820 g to 2,500 g or moderate anomalies; and group C has a birthweight of less than 1,820 g or severe anomalies. Short-term mortality is approximately 0% for group A infants, 5% for group B infants, and 34% for group C infants.[116,117,118,119] The most common complications following surgery include stricture or leakage at the attachment site and reflux of stomach contents into the esophagus. Strictures occur in as many as 40% of patients but usually can be corrected by mechanical dilation.[120,121] Anastomotic leaks are potentially serious but are less common and typically resolve over time. Reflux may lead to recurrent pneumonia and broncho-spasm;[122,123] as many as 70% of affected children undergo surgery (fundoplication) to halt this process.

Congenital Diaphragmatic Hernia

Congenital diaphragmatic hernia (CDH) is characterized by abnormal fusion of the diaphragm during fetal development, with herniation of abdominal organs into the thorax. Depending on the location of the defect, the stomach, small intestine, liver, spleen, colon, or pancreas may be involved. Defects of the lateral portion (posterolateral) of the diaphragm make up 85% to 90% of cases of CDH,[124] are usually evident during the first few days of life, and are accompanied by respiratory distress due to inadequate lung development. Approximately 5% of cases become manifest after the neonatal period.[125] Defects of the diaphragm behind the breastbone (retrosternal) occur less often and are more benign. These hernias usually manifest with signs of bowel obstruction rather than respiratory distress.[126] A third type of CDH is known as an eventration, which is characterized by normal fusion but deficient muscular development of the diaphragm. Eventrations allow abdominal organs to protrude, but not herniate, into the thorax. The etiology of CDH is unknown.

In posterolateral defects, the pulmonary artery pressure does not drop as it normally should after birth because low oxygen levels in the blood and acidosis stimulate constriction of the muscle fibers that surround small arteries in the lungs. Desaturated blood is then shunted across the foramen ovale (an abnormally persistent opening between the left and right atria) or ductus arteriosus (an abnormally persistent connection between the aorta and the main pulmonary artery), bypassing the lungs. Without prompt surgery, failure of blood flow to vital organs (ischemia), shock, and death rapidly ensue. Associated anomalies may include malrotation of the intestine, chest enlargement,[127] and underdevelopment of the left ventricle.[128] Malformations of the cardiovascular, genitourinary, central nervous, or musculoskeletal systems occur in 17%[129] to 40% of cases.[130]

Surgical management of CDH involves rapidly closing the diaphragmatic defect and restoring herniated abdominal organs to their normal positions. Large defects are closed by inserting a prosthesis or transferring a muscle flap from the abdominal wall.[131] Postoperative mortality of approximately 50% was reported in the 1970s and early 1980s[132,133,134] but has decreased to 25% to 30% since the introduction of extracorporeal membrane oxygenation

(ECMO).[135] ECMO is a technique for oxygenating venous blood outside the body and returning it to the systemic circulation. Complications of its use include stroke, infection, and anticoagulant-related hemorrhage. Long-term follow-up studies of children with CDH have noted abnormalities in lung ventilation and perfusion,[136,137] exercise intolerance, and wheezing.[138] Esophageal abnormalities, reflux of stomach contents into the esophagus, and fibrous adhesions surrounding the intestines also have been reported.[139] These conditions may interfere with weight gain but usually improve with supportive care.

Eventration of the diaphragm is corrected by focal resection or plication of the maldeveloped portion. In mild cases, continuous positive airway pressure through the nose, applied for several months, may support the diaphragm and obviate the need for surgery.

Intestinal Atresia or Stenosis: Duodenal Atresia

The duodenum is the first and shortest portion of the small intestine. Duodenal atresia typically manifests with the vomiting of bilious fluid, abdominal distention, and dehydration. It results from failure of the embryonic intestinal tube to recanalize. This defect often is associated with prematurity (35% to 60% of cases),[140,141,142] Down syndrome (up to 44% of cases),[143] or both. Between 30% and 60% of affected children have other anomalies such as congenital heart defects, a ring-shaped pancreas, malrotation of the intestines, esophageal atresia, and an imperforate anus.[144,145] Without surgery, all intestinal atresias are fatal.

In most patients, the closed (atretic) duodenal segment can be resected and the normal segments of intestine on either side can be surgically attached (anastamosed). If the duodenum is narrowed but patent, excision of the obstructive web without resection is preferable. In the largest recent series, operative mortality was 3% and late postoperative mortality was 9%, with most deaths resulting from congenital heart disease. In less than 20% of patients, another operation may be necessary for malfunction or perforation of the anastomosis, overlooked stenoses elsewhere, or adhesions. Children who survive the neonatal period do exceedingly well, but some patients experience reflux of stomach contents into the esophagus or impaired intestinal function.

Intestinal Atresia or Stenosis: Jejunoileal Atresia

The jejunum and ileum are the second and third portions of the small intestine, respectively. Jejunoileal atresia also manifests with vomiting of bilious fluid and abdominal distention. Multiple segments of the jejunum are involved in 15% to 30% of cases.[146] Jejunoileal atresia is believed to result from insufficient blood supply to the fetal intestine and is associated with prematurity in 40% to 60% of cases[147] and cystic fibrosis in 10% to 20% of cases. "Apple peel atresia" is a particularly severe form of the defect caused by obstruction of the superior mesenteric artery, which supplies blood to most of the small intestine, with compensatory overgrowth of viable small intestine.[148] Associated anomalies outside the gastrointestinal tract are unusual. Associated gastrointestinal anomalies may include malrotation, twisting or perforation of the intestine, and gastroschisis (see below).

Most infants with jejunoileal atresia undergo resection of the atretic segment of intestine, with anastamosis of the normal segments on either side. In difficult cases, it is sometimes necessary to bring both segments of intestine to the skin and reconnect them several months later. Intravenous nutrition is an important component of these infants' care after surgery. Several recent studies neglected to distinguish between early and late deaths, but the average total mortality was 10%.[149] In most cases, death was attributable to failure of the anastomosis, sepsis, abdominal abscess, or liver failure related to intravenous nutrition. Complications arising soon after surgery include obstruction or necrotizing infection of the intestine, and infections of other sites. Complications arising later such as chronic diarrhea, failure to thrive, malabsorption of nutrients due to "short gut," and secondary bowel obstruction are reported in approximately 27% of cases.

Intestinal Atresia or Stenosis: Colonic Atresia

Fewer infants are born with atresia of the colon than with atresia of the small intestine. Colonic atresia usually manifests with the infant's failing to pass stool and having abdominal distention. The infant also may have vomiting and a palpable abdominal mass. The etiology of this disorder is presumed to be ischemic, that is, related to insufficient blood flow to the fetal colon.[150] In several reported cases, colonic atresia has been associated with gastroschisis, jejunoileal atresia, or anomalies outside the gastrointestinal tract.[151]

Most infants with colonic atresia undergo resection of the atretic segment of large intestine, with anastamosis of the normal segments on either side. In difficult cases, it is sometimes necessary to bring both segments of intestine to the skin (e.g., colostomy) and reconnect them several months later. Mortality associated with this surgery in three recent series averaged 12%.[152] Most of the children who died had serious associated anomalies. Complications of surgery include narrowing at the anastamotic site, secondary bowel obstruction, and colostomy dysfunction.

Intestinal Atresia or Stenosis: Anorectal Malformations

Anorectal malformations are classified by the anatomic level at which they occur: the rectum ends above the levator ani muscle in "high atresias" and below it in "low atresias."[153] This muscle helps maintain fecal continence. Anorectal malformations usually manifest with failure to pass stool and an abnormally small, absent, or misplaced anal opening.[154,155] Approximately 75% to 80% of children with anorectal atresia have an abnormal channel (fistula) between the rectum or anus and the bladder, urethra, vagina, scrotum, or skin.[156,157] Fistulas to the urinary tract predispose the infant to recurrent bladder and kidney infections. High atresias are associated with malformations outside the gastrointestinal tract[158] such as the VATER or VACTERL syndrome, which includes vertebral, anal, cardiac, tracheoesophageal, renal, and limb defects.[159]

The repair of low atresias involves serial dilations of the affected area or surgical reconstruction, with or without transplantation of the anus. Most surgeons perform a temporary colostomy when the child has a high atresia, then pull the intact colon down to form a new anus several months to two years later. Mortality of 15% to 20% has been reported, although most of these deaths are attributable to associated anomalies.[160,161,162,163]   Complications occur after surgery in 25% to 40% of cases.[164,165]   They include narrowing of the anal canal, prolapse of rectal mucosa through the anus, obstruction of the intestine by fibrous adhesions, and recurrent fistulas. These complications often necessitate repeat surgery to dilate the anus, resect prolapsed mucous membranes, or lyse adhesions. Long-term follow-up studies suggest that as many as 50% of infants surviving a high atresia suffer from fecal incontinence, as compared with fewer than 10% of those surviving a low atresia.[166,167,168]   Muscle-transfer surgery and special training may improve continence.

Renal Agenesis, Hypoplasia, or Dysgenesis

Developmental abnormalities of the kidney include its absence (agenesis), underdevelopment (hypoplasia), improper development (dysgenesis), and cystic replacement. We did not study cystic kidney disease because the most commonly used disease classification system in the United States, ICD-9-CM, does not distinguish between the autosomal recessive and autosomal dominant types. As these names suggest, the two types have different mechanisms of inheritance; only the the autosomal recessive type appears in infants.

Bilateral renal agenesis (Potter syndrome),[169] affecting both kidneys, results from defective development of an embryonic structure called the ureteral bud. It causes a severe deficiency of amniotic fluid (oligohydramnios) that, in turn, causes poor fetal growth, an abnormal face, misshapen ears, limb abnormalities, and underdevelopment of the lungs.[170] These children usually die within several weeks of birth from breathing problems and kidney failure. Surgery is not indicated, and generally only supportive care is provided.

In cases of unilateral renal agenesis, the solitary kidney compensates by becoming larger than normal; it often may be felt as an abdominal mass. Some patients with this disorder remain free of symptoms throughout life, whereas others develop thickening of important membranes in the kidney, spill protein in the urine, and, ultimately experience kidney failure because of increased blood flow through the solitary kidney.[171,172] Unilateral renal agenesis may be associated with a ventricular septal defect, spina bifida, gastrointestinal anomalies, or skeletal anomalies.[173] The natural history of this defect is obscure because asymptomatic cases were not diagnosed before prenatal ultrasound became widely used. However, these patients probably have an increased likelihood of developing hypertension, urinary tract infections, and kidney stones.

Renal hypoplasia is characterized by small kidneys that have a deficient number of nephrons (functioning units) or nephrons of abnormally small size. If both kidneys are underdeveloped, the nephrons generally are reduced in number but markedly enlarged. Children with this defect have an impaired ability to concentrate urine, which causes frequent voiding and recurrent dehydration. They also excrete excessive amounts of sodium and protein. Kidney function may be stable for the first several years of life, but progressive deposits in the kidneys' filtration system and fibrosis lead to kidney failure after an average interval of seven years. Kidney dialysis becomes necessary within one to two years after chronic kidney failure is first diagnosed.[174]

Renal dysplasia is characterized by abnormal differentiation of important structures in the kidney during fetal development. The glomeruli, tubules, and ducts look disorganized and primitive, and the kidneys' excretory function is poor. Dysplastic kidneys include a mixture of embryonic elements (e.g., cartilage, bone, and fibrous tissue), and cysts are a common feature. Two forms of cystic dysplasia have been described: small cystic kidneys often are associated with defects of the opposite kidney, whereas large cystic kidneys are not.[175] Nearly all children with renal dysplasia have associated urinary tract anomalies such as absence or narrowing of the ureter, which occurs with unilateral dysplasia, and posterior urethral valves, which occur with bilateral dysplasia.[176] Indeed, experimental studies suggest that ureteral obstruction may be the primary cause of cystic dysplasia.[177,178]

Renal dysplasia involving both kidneys manifests similarly to Potter syndrome, with a deficiency of amniotic fluid (oligohydramnios) and underdevelopment of the lungs. It progresses quickly to chronic kidney failure and death. Approximately 50% of children with unilateral cystic dysplasia are noted to have a palpable abdominal mass.[179,180]   Other symptoms include failure to thrive, urinary tract infection, and unrelated anomalies.   Renal cell carcinoma,[181,182] Wilms tumor,[183] and nodular renal blastema (a precursor of Wilms tumor)[184] have been reported to arise in dysplastic kidneys, suggesting that prophylactic resection may be appropriate. However, cystic kidneys detected by ultrasound may regress   spontaneously,   even   after   birth.[185,186,187]   Many urologists, therefore, recommend resection only if the involved kidney continues to enlarge or causes hypertension.[188]

Congenital Urinary Tract Obstruction

Congenital obstruction of the urinary tract generally occurs at the junction between the pelvis of the kidney and the ureter (ureteropelvic junction) or the junction between the ureter and the bladder (ureterovesical junction). Ureteropelvic junction (UPJ) obstruction causes congenital distention of the kidney's urinary collecting system.[189,190]   Most cases are detected by prenatal ultrasonography; the remaining cases come to medical attention with a palpable flank mass, urinary tract infection, or associated anomalies.[191,192]   Oligohydramnios and underdevelopment of the lungs may affect the fetus with bilateral UPJ obstruction.[193]   UPJ obstruction generally results from abnormal organization of the muscle fibers that control the ureter's rhythmic contractions, or peristalsis. Less common causes include extrinsic compression by an abnormally placed artery or fibrous adhesions and polyps or mucosal folds within the ureter. Serial ultrasonography has shown that as many as 40% of UPJ obstructions diagnosed before birth resolve spontaneously,[194] but others progress to kidney failure if surgery is not performed.

The current medical practice is to assess kidney function during the neonatal period; children with impaired function undergo reconstruction of the origin of the ureter (pyeloplasty) soon after birth to correct the obstruction and to prevent further deterioration.[195,196]   Children with normal or equivocal function have serial follow-up evaluations with ultrasound and often require pyeloplasty later.[197,198]   Approximately 90% of newborn infants who undergo pyeloplasty have a satisfactory outcome, with reduced dilation of the urinary collecting system and improved or maintained kidney function.[199,200]   Complications of surgery include leakage at the ureteropelvic anastomosis, recurrent obstruction, and infection. High-risk patients may undergo ureteropyelotomy performed using a new, less invasive endoscopic technique.[201]   Between 7% and 21% of children who have UPJ obstruction have coexisting reflux of urine from the bladder to the ureter (vesicoureteral reflux), which may be treated prophylactically with antibiotics and/or reimplantation of the ureter.[202]

Ureterovesical junction (UVJ) obstruction causes congenital distention of the ureter.   Most cases are detected by prenatal ultrasonography; the remaining cases come to medical attention with a palpable flank mass, urinary tract infection, or associated anomalies. These anomalies include vesicoureteral reflux, which occurs in as many as 20% of cases,[203] UPJ obstruction, cystic renal dysplasia, and duplication of the ureter.   UVJ obstruction resembles UPJ obstruction; that is, it generally results from ineffective rhythmic contractions (peristalsis), but less common causes include extrinsic compression by an overlying vessel or pelvic mass.   Many children with mild hydroureter and good kidney function can be managed without surgery.   These children receive periodic follow-up evaluations to detect early signs of deteriorating kidney function.[204]

When surgery is necessary, the preferred approach is primary reconstruction, which involves resecting the abnormal segment of ureter and reimplanting the ureter into the bladder.   Because the ureter usually is dilated, plication or tapering of the end to be implanted may be necessary.[205]   Temporary diversion of the ureter to the abdominal wall (ureterostomy), with delayed reconstruction, is an approach reserved for children who have a massively dilated ureter, poor kidney function, or severe coexisting illness. Complications after surgery occur in 10% of cases or less but include stricture at the new anastomosis, vesicoureteral reflux, and iatrogenic injury to the ureter or bladder.   Both UPJ and UVJ obstruction can progress to end-stage kidney disease, even after a timely surgical repair.[206]

Congenital Limb Reduction

Congenital limb reduction is characterized by the partial or complete absence of upper- or lower-limb bones, with or without the involvement of other tissues. One widely used classification system[207,208] categorizes limb reductions as amelias, in which an entire limb is absent, or meromelias, in which only a portion of the limb is absent. Meromelias are further categorized as terminal or intercalary defects. In terminal defects, all bones beyond the deficiency are affected. Intercalary defects are characterized by intact structures beyond the defect but partial or total absence of bones closer to the trunk. Both of these types are further subclassified as transverse, if the defect affects the complete width of a limb, or longitudinal, if it extends down the long axis of a limb. Transverse defects are further defined by the level at which the limb terminates.[209] Approximately 2% of congenital limb reductions are amelias, 26% are terminal transverse defects, 48% are terminal longitudinal defects, and 23% are intercalary defects. Reduction defects affect upper limbs alone (68%) more often than lower limbs alone (23%) or upper and lower limbs (9%).[210] Defects on the right and left side are almost equally common; approximately 14% of patients have symmetric bilateral defects. Longitudinal defects of the arm most commonly involve the radius or bones of the wrist, and longitudinal defects of the leg most commonly involve the fibula. Transverse defects of the arm most often occur below the elbow or at the wrist; transverse defects of the leg are unusual.[211,212,213]

Limb reductions reflect abnormal development of embryonic limb buds. Teratogens such as thalidomide are responsible for some cases, but for most the cause is still unknown. Associated malformations occur in 30% to 53% of affected children,[214,215] including heart and kidney anomalies, imperforate anus, esophageal atresia, omphalocele (an abdominal wall defect described below), spina bifida, vertebral anomalies, webbing between the fingers or toes, and cleft palate. Limb deficiencies are seen in many multidefect syndromes such as the VATER association described earlier.[216] Between 12% and 20% of infants with limb reductions die during infancy; approximately 85% of these deaths are attributable to other anomalies. Fewer than 50% of infants with amelia survive.[217]

The treatment of congenital limb reductions involves fitting appropriate prostheses, providing physical and occupational therapy, and performing surgery to improve appearance or function. Upper-limb prostheses are designed to provide a grip mechanism and to permit effective bimanual coordination. Infants typically are fitted with passive prostheses that parents can manipulate, whereas older children are fitted with cable-operated or electrically powered prostheses. Lower-limb prostheses are designed to foster maneuverability by equalizing leg length, correcting malrotation, and improving stability.[218] Prostheses generally must be replaced annually until the child is five years of age, then every other year until twelve years of age, and then every two to five years throughout life. Most children with leg prostheses walk well, although often with a longer stride length and slower cadence than normal children.[219] Despite these efforts, affected children have permanent disabilities with significant psychosocial implications.

Certain reduction defects raise special treatment issues. Congenital deficiency of the fibula leads to a shortened leg and an outwardly angulated foot,[220] which interfere with normal gait and preclude fitting a suitable prosthesis. For this reason, most orthopedic surgeons recommend amputating the foot (while preserving the heel pad) before a child starts school, unless his or her legs are relatively similar in length.[221] Modest discrepancies can be corrected by lengthening the tibia and/or the femur, fusing growth plates in the opposite leg, or reconstructing the ankle.[222] Complications of amputation are rare, although skin breakdown and migration of the heel pad have been reported.[223,224,225,226]

Congenital deficiency of the tibia leads to a shortened and bowed leg, an unstable knee joint, and an inwardly angulated foot.[227] The tibia may be completely absent, with or without a normal growth plate at the end of the femur, or simply undeveloped at the upper or lower end.[228] Surgical options include transposing the fibula to articulate directly with the femur,[229] disarticulating the knee and amputating the lower leg, and fusing the upper tibial fragment to the intact fibula or lower femur.[230,231,232]

Congenital deficiency of the femur may be separated into two subgroups: underdevelopment (hypoplasia) and focal deficiency of the upper (proximal) femur.[233] Because hypoplasia usually is associated with a stable hip joint, the primary goal of therapy is to equalize leg length by lengthening the femur or fusing growth plates in the opposite femur. Potential complications of the former procedure include partial dislocation of the knee and fracture of the lengthened bone. The goals of therapy for proximal focal femoral deficiency include equalizing leg length and stabilizing the hip joint, thus avoiding hip contractures that would interfere with mobility.[234] These goals may be achieved by performing one or more of several procedures such as fusing the tibia to the femur, amputating the foot to facilitate fitting an extension prosthesis, removing a segment of femur on the normal side, and rotating the tibia to convert the ankle joint into a knee joint. Potential complications of this rotation-plasty include derotation of the tibia and poor function.[235]

Surgical therapy of upper-limb deficiencies often is less necessary because weight-bearing is not an issue. One exception is congenital deficiency of the radius, which is characterized by a short, bowed forearm with an outwardly deviated hand. Hand function can be improved by transposing the ulna and fusing the wrist.[236] If the thumb is absent, a functional thumb can be created from an index finger or a transplanted toe. Bone-lengthening procedures may benefit children with underdeveloped fingers. Children with bilateral hand reductions may undergo a procedure to split the forearm stumps into forceps that can be used to grasp objects.[237]

Abdominal Wall Defects: Gastroschisis and Omphalocele

Gastroschisis and omphalocele are defects of the abdominal wall.[238] In gastroschisis, the defect is located to the right of an intact navel and permits extrusion of abdominal contents. The defect in omphalocele is within the umbilical ring; herniating abdominal contents are surrounded by an intact or ruptured sac. Bowel swelling and necrosis are more common with gastroschisis, perhaps because this defect tends to be smaller[239] and the herniated bowel is in direct contact with amniotic fluid.[240] Gastroschisis may originate from obstruction of the right umbilical vein. By contrast, approximately 50% of fetuses with omphalocele diagnosed by ultrasound have chromosomal abnormalities such as trisomy 18;[241] many of these pregnancies end in spontaneous or elective abortions. Omphalocele is also a component of several multidefect syndromes.[242]

Intestinal atresia is noted in 7% to 30% of infants with gastroschisis, presumably because an associated volvulus (twisting) or tight abdominal wall defect compromises blood flow to the developing intestine.[243] However, associated anomalies involving the intestines, heart (e.g., tetralogy of Fallot, septal defects[244]), diaphragm, and genitourinary tract are more common with omphalocele (33% to 56%) than with gastroschisis (5% to 20%).[245,246,247,248,249] The size of the omphalocele is associated with the prevalence of major malformations and the risk of death.[250] The prognosis for both defects is poor unless they are treated surgically.

Because many cases of gastroschisis currently are diagnosed in the womb by serum alpha fetoprotein testing and ultrasound, the treatment of this disorder begins before the child is born. Some physicians argue that an affected fetus should be delivered by cesarean section because uterine contractions and vaginal delivery may damage herniated viscera and compromise their blood supply.[251,252] However, infants delivered vaginally do not consistently show worse outcomes than those delivered by cesarean section.[253,254,255,256] Surgical closure of gastroschisis is best performed within six hours after the infant's birth in order to minimize the risks of hypothermia, dehydration, and infection. Primary closure can be achieved in 75% to 85% of patients. The remainder requires construction of a temporary Silastic "chimney" to accommodate the herniated organs, followed by definitive closure several days later.[257] Segments of intestine that are atretic, narrowed, or gangrenous are resected. Postoperative care includes intravenous fluids, antibiotics, and nutrition for one to four weeks. In recent series, mortality during and after surgery was less than 10%.[258,259,260,261,262,263,264] Complications of surgery such as infections of the wound or blood, prolonged dysfunction or obstruction of the intestines, malabsorption of nutrients due to "short gut," abnormal connections between the intestine and the skin (enterocutaneous fistulae), and intestinal necrosis or injury occur in as many as 42% of cases.[265] Necrotizing enterocolitis, a life-threatening infection of the intestinal lining, may develop as long as thirty to sixty days after gastroschisis repair.[266]

Surgical closure of omphalocele is not as urgent as is the closure of gastroschisis because the peritoneal sac reduces the risk of infection and dehydration and because evaluation of associated anomalies may affect decisions about therapy. Children with trisomy 18 or other fatal anomalies may be allowed to die without surgery or may undergo palliative "painting" of the sac with a chemical that causes tissue destruction. Small omphaloceles are repaired by primary closure. For giant omphaloceles, it generally is necessary to reduce the defect in serial operations over a one-week period using a prosthetic pouch. Mortality among infants with omphalocele has varied from 19% to 29% in recent series, but the percentage depends primarily on whether associated anomalies exist. Complications after surgery are less frequent than after gastroschisis repair because failure of blood flow to the bowel and bowel necrosis occur less frequently.

Long-term follow-up studies of children born with abdominal wall defects show normal intestinal function and fat absorption,[267] poor weight gain during the first one to three years of life,[268] and subsequent normalization of height and weight.[269] A small percentage of children require reoperation to reduce the reflux of stomach acid into the esophagus or treat intestinal obstruction. Approximately 18% of survivors in one study demonstrated behavioral problems, although their intellectual ability was normal.[270]

Down Syndrome

Trisomy 21, Down syndrome, is the most common congenital malformation syndrome. Affected infants have poor muscle tone, increased joint flexibility, folds of redundant skin on the back of the neck, a flat bridge of the nose, upslanting eyelid fissures, small or anomalous ears, an abnormally developed pelvis, unusually small middle phalanges in the fifth fingers and toes, and "simian" hand creases.[271] Other physical signs include an unusually small head (in 50% of cases), "mongolian" skin folds along the inner aspects of the upper eyelids (50% to 70%), speckled irides in both eyes (30% to 80%), a narrow and short palate (60% to 90%), a protruding tongue (40% to 60%), broad hands (70%), wide spaces between the first two toes (50% to 90%), a vertical lower lip crease (50%), and prominent sole creases (65%).[272] The most significant associated anomalies are cardiac; 29% of children with Down syndrome in four population registries were diagnosed with congenital heart disease (CHD).[273,274,275,276]   Atrioventricular canal (in 24% to 61% of those with CHD) and ventricular septal defects (in 16% to 33%) are the most common cardiac anomalies.[277,278,279]   Duodenal atresia or stenosis occurs in 2.6% of children born with Down syndrome.[280] Other associated anomalies include tracheoesophageal fistula, imperforate anus,[281] cleft lip or palate, fused digits, congenital cataracts,[282] failure of the testicles to descend to the scrotum, and incomplete development of neck vertebrae.[283]

Approximately 95% of Down syndrome cases result from the failure of chromosome 21 to separate normally (nondisjunction), leading one ovum or sperm cell to receive an extra copy of the chromosome. The likelihood of nondisjunction increases with the mother's age.[284] Most other cases of Down syndrome result from translocation of part of chromosome 21 onto another chromosome. Mothers who are carriers of this translocation may transmit the defect (or the asymptomatic carrier condition) to their children.

A variety of health problems affects persons with Down syndrome. Approximately 14% are mildly mentally retarded, 55% are moderately retarded, 22% to 27% are severely retarded, and 3% to 12% are profoundly retarded.[285,286]   Among the profoundly retarded, 15% are unable to walk, 16% are unable to feed themselves, and 3% require feeding through a tube. In cross-sectional studies, 5% to 10% of persons with Down syndrome have decreased thyroid function and more than 10% have decreased thyroid responsiveness to pituitary regulation.[287,288,289,290,291] Laxity of the ligaments causes unusual flexibility and degenerative changes in many joints, including the knees[292] and spine.[293] Approximately 10% to 15% of children with Down syndrome show evidence of instability between the first two neck vertebrae,[294,295] although the risk of subsequent dislocation at this site is unknown.[296] Approximately 50% of asymptomatic adolescents and adults have a benign heart condition called mitral valve prolapse, and 10% have backward flow across the aortic valve.[297,298] Approximately 60% of children with Down syndrome have hearing loss caused by chronic middle ear disease; 15% to 26% have moderate, severe, or profound hearing loss.[299,300,301]   Antibiotics and pressure-equalization tubes often are used as therapy but may not be effective.[302]   Eye abnormalities associated with Down syndrome[303] include premature cataracts (12% to 20%), strabismus (20% to 45%), severe nearsightedness, and a conical deformity of the cornea called keratoconus.[304,305,306,307,308] Approximately 5% to 9% of Down syndrome patients experience seizures[309,310,311,312,313,314,315]; this prevalence increases with age.[316]   Other associated health problems include obesity, obstruction of the airway during sleep[317,318] and gum disease.[319] An increased risk of skin and lung infections presumably is attributable to impaired immune function.[320]   Finally, Down syndrome increases the risk of acute leukemia twelvefold.[321,322,323,324]   Among patients with one type of leukemia, those with Down syndrome are less likely to respond to chemotherapy (81% versus 94%),[325] develop more side effects on therapy,[326] and have worse five-year survival (28% versus 59%)[327] than patients who have normal chromosomes.

All of these health problems are treated with medications, surgery, and prosthetic devices such as hearing aids, as appropriate. Children with Down syndrome who have associated cardiac or gastrointestinal anomalies are treated in the same manner as children with normal chromosomes.   Nonetheless, most persons with Down syndrome experience memory loss and other signs of progressive cognitive impairment after forty-five years of age.[328,329,330,331]   Autopsy studies show pathologic changes resembling Alzheimer's disease in the brains of persons with Down syndrome,[332,333]   although differences in brain metabolism have been identified.[334]

Cerebral Palsy

Cerebral palsy is a chronic, nonprogressive disorder of movement or posture that becomes manifest during early childhood.[335]   This definition excludes disorders that arise after serious trauma or infection. Several subtypes of cerebral palsy have been recognized. Spastic cerebral palsy is characterized by weakness, increased muscle tone, exaggerated reflexes, and a proclivity to joint contractures. The spasticity may affect all four extremities equally (quadriplegia) or may affect the legs more than the arms (diplegia). Alternatively, the spasticity may affect only the legs (paraplegia), an arm and leg on the same side (hemiplegia), or one extremity alone (monoplegia).

Athetoid cerebral palsy is characterized by uncontrolled and uncoordinated movements, which are often intensified by stress and voluntary activity. Ataxic cerebral palsy is characterized by a wide-based gait and difficulty performing repetitive movements; this form of cerebral palsy has the best prognosis. Approximately 70% of children with cerebral palsy are classified as spastic, whereas 15% are athetotic, 5% are ataxic, and the remainder have a mixed disorder.[336] Even though 21% of children with cerebral palsy have a major malformation not involving the central nervous system, no specific defects predominate.

The etiology of cerebral palsy involves many factors and is poorly understood.[337] Known risk factors include low birthweight, major malformations not involving the central nervous system, breech presentation at birth, a mentally retarded mother,[338] low placental weight, premature separation of the placenta, and an unusually long or short interval between pregnancies.[339] No more than one third of children with spastic cerebral palsy have a history of asphyxia,[340,341] and only 14% of cases are clearly attributable to that cause.[342] Despite major changes in obstetric management, the incidence of cerebral palsy among infants of normal birthweight did not change significantly between the 1960s and the 1980s.[343,344,345]

Associated impairments are related to the severity and type of cerebral palsy. Between 22% and 50% of children with cerebral palsy develop epilepsy.[346,347,348,349,350] This percentage is 33% to 40% among children with hemiplegic cerebral palsy[351,352] but exceeds 90% among those with quadriplegic cerebral palsy.[353] Between 25% and 35% of children with cerebral palsy have normal intelligence (IQ ≥ 86 or ≥ 90), but approximately 25% have severe or profound retardation (IQ ≤ 35).[354,355] The latter percentage varies from 5% among persons with mild to moderate cerebral palsy to 65% among those with severe cerebral palsy (who have appliance-limited function or no function in their affected limbs).[356] Virtually all children with quadriplegic cerebral palsy are severely retarded. Children with cerebral palsy also may have severe hearing deficits (approximately 5% overall but more frequent with athetoid cerebral palsy[357,358,359]), visual deficits (7% to 20%), strabismus, speech disorders, poorly developed enamel on the primary teeth,[360] hip dislocation, and curvature of the spine.[361]

The treatment of cerebral palsy is designed to optimize functional status and to minimize disability. Even though various "neuromotor" therapies have been promoted,[362] the evidence supporting their effectiveness is weak.[363,364,365,366,367]   Adaptive devices (e.g., wheelchairs or walkers) and tone-inhibiting casts or splints may be useful.[368,369]   Severe spasticity may be treated with medications.[370,371]   In order to restore balance between opposing muscle groups, orthopedic surgeons may elongate or transfer tendons, divide spastic muscles or tendons, release tight bands of connective tissue, fuse joints, cut nerves that supply spastic muscles, or resect pieces of bone.[372,373,374]   Selective posterior rhizotomy is a neurosurgical procedure designed to reduce spasticity by carefully dividing sensory nerve roots.[375]   Even though this procedure may benefit carefully selected patients,[376,377] it remains controversial because of serious complications that include loss of sensation and decreased muscle tone.[378]   The evaluation of new therapies is complicated by the variable course of cerebral palsy and the possibility of spontaneous remission.[379,380]

The survival and functional outcomes of children with cerebral palsy are highly correlated with their intellectual level. Survival to twenty years of age is essentially normal among persons with $IQ \geq 50$ (98%) but is substantially less (72%) among those with lower IQs.[381]   Similar differences have been reported in relation to manual dexterity and walking ability. Among adults of normal intelligence ($IQ \geq 80$) with cerebral palsy, 39% are independent and 48% are partially dependent; this compares with 1% and 17%, respectively, among those of lower intelligence.[382]   Many adults with cerebral palsy require sheltered living or work environments,[383] although predictions of future needs made during childhood are often incorrect.[384]   Female adolescents with cerebral palsy have lower self-esteem than those without cerebral palsy.[385]   Adolescents with cerebral palsy may have difficulty with heterosexual relationships.[386]

Endnotes to Appendix 1

1.Myrianthopoulos NC, Melnick M. Studies in neural tube defects. I. epidemiologic and etiologic aspects. *Am J Med Genet.* 1987;26:783-796.

2.Mulinare J, Cordero JF, Erickson JD, Berry RJ. Periconceptional use of multivitamins and the occurrence of neural tube defects. *JAMA.* 1988;260:3141-3145.

3.Mills JL, Rhoads GG, Simpson JL, Cunningham GC, Conley MR, Lassman MR, et al. The absence of a relation between the periconceptional use of vitamins and neural tube defects. *New Engl J Med.* 1989;321:430-435.

4.Bower C, Stanley FJ. Dietary folate as a risk factor for neural-tube defects: evidence from a case-control study in Western Australia. *Med J Aust.* 1989;150:613-619.

5.Milunsky A, Jick H, Jick SS, Bruell CL, MacLaughlin DS, Rothman KJ, Willett W. Multivitamin/folic acid supplementation in early pregnancy reduces the prevalence of neural tube defects. *JAMA.* 1989;262:2847-2852.

6.McBride ML. Sib risks of anencephaly and spina bifida in British Columbia. *Am J Med Genet.* 1979;3:377-387.

7.Stone DH. The declining prevalence of anencephalus and spina bifida: its nature, causes and implications. *Develop Med Child Neurol.* 1987;29:541-549.

8.Lorber J, Ward AM. Spina bifida-a vanishing nightmare? *Arch Dis Child.* 1985;60:1086-1091.

9.Laurence KM. A declining incidence of neural tube defects in the UK. *Z Kinderchir.* 1989;44(suppl I):51.

10.Wiswell TE, Tuttle DJ, Northam RS, Simonds GR. Major congenital neurologic malformations: a 17-year survey. *AJDC.* 1990;144:61-67.

11.Bamforth SJ, Baird PA. Spina bifida and hydrocephalus: a population study over a 35-year period. *Am J Hum Genet.* 1989;44:225-232.

12.Gaston H. Does the spina bifida clinic need an ophthalmologist? *Z Kinderchir.* 1985;40(suppl I):46-50.

13.Bartoshesky LE, Haller J, Scott RM, Wojick C. Seizures in children with meningomyelocele. *AJDC.* 1985;139:400-402.

14.Hosking GP. Fits in hydrocephalic children. *Arch Dis Child.* 1974;49:633.

15.Hunt GM. Spina bifida: implications for 100 children at school. *Develop Med Child Neurol.* 1981;23:160-172.

16.Samuelsson L, Eklof O. Scoliosis in myelomeningocele. *Acta Orthop Scand.* 1988;59(2):122-127.

17.Shurtleff DB, Gordon LH, Goiney R, et al. Myelodysplasia: the natural history of kyphosis and scoliosis-A preliminary report. *Dev Med Child Neurol.* 1976;18(suppl 377):126-133.

18.Jacobs RA, Wolfe G, Rasmuson M. Upper extremity dysfunction in children with myelomeningocele. *Z Kinderchir.* 1988;43(suppl II):19-21.

19.Turner A. Upper limb functioning of children with myelomeningocele. *Dev Med Child Neurol.* 1986;28:790-798.

20.Thomas AP, Bax MCO, Smyth DPL. The health care of physically handicapped young adults. *Z Kinderchir.* 1987;42(suppl I):57-59.

21.Blum RW, Resnick MD, Nelson R, St Germaine A. Family and peer issues among adolescents with spina bifida and cerebral palsy. *Pediatrics.* 1992; 88:280-285.

22.Tew B, Laurence KM, Jenins V. Factors affecting employability among young adults with spina bifida and hydrocephalus. *Z Kinderchir.* 1990;45(suppl I):34-36.

23.McLone DG. Results of treatment of children born with a myelomeningocele. *Clinical Neurosurgery.* 1983;30:407-412.

24.Luthy DA, Wardinsky T, Shurtleff DB, Hollenbach KA, Hickok DE, Nyberg DA, et al. Cesarean section before the onset of labor and subsequent motor function in infants with meningomyelocele diagnosed antenatally. *New Engl J Med.* 1991;324:662-666.

25.Bensen JT, Dillard RG, Burton BK. Open spina bifida: does cesarean section delivery improve prognosis? *Obstet Gynecol.* 1988;71:532-534.

26.Sharrard WJW, Zachary RB, Lorber J, Bruce AM. A controlled trial of immediate and delayed closure of spina bifida cystica. *Arch Dis Child.* 1963;38:18-22.

27.Guiney EJ, Fitzgerald RJ, Goldberg C. A review of the management policy for newborn spina bifida children at Our Lady's Hospital for Sick Children, Crumlin, 1973-1983. *Z Kinderchir.* 1984;39(suppl II):114-116.

28.Guiney EJ, Fitzgerald RJ, Blake NS, Goldberg C. Status of a group of spina bifida children not managed by early surgery. *Z Kinderchir.* 1986;41(suppl I):16-17.

29.Gross RH, Cox A, Tatyrek R, Pollay M, Barnes WA. Early management and decision making for the treatment of myelomeningocele. *Pediatrics.* 1983;72:450-458.

30.McLaughlin JF, Shurtleff DB, Lamers JY, Stuntz JT, Hayden PW, Kropp RJ. Influence of prognosis on decisions regarding the care of newborns with myelodysplasia. *New Engl J Med.* 1985;312:1589-1594.

31.Beeger JH, Meihuizen de Regt MJ, HogenEsch I, Ter Weeme CA, Mooij JJA, Vencken LM. Progressive neurologic deficit in children with spina bifida aperta. *Z Kinderchir.* 1986;41(suppl I):13-15.

32.Beeger JH, Wiertsema GPA, Breukers SME, Mooy JJA, Ter Weeme CA. Tethered cord syndrome: clinical signs and results of operation in 42 patients with spina bifida aperta and occulta. *Z Kinderchir.* 1989;44(suppl I):5-7.

33.Tamaki N, Shirataki K, Kojima N, et al. Tethered cord syndrome of delayed onset following repair of myelomeningocele. *J Neurosurg.* 1988;69:393-398.

34.Sherk HH, Pasquariello PS, Charney E, Schut L. Central nervous system lesions and developmental scoliosis in myelomeningocele. *Z Kinderchir.* 1983;38(suppl II):87-89.

35.Lorber J, Lyons VH. Arterial hypertension in children with spina bifida cystica and urinary incontinence. *Develop Med Child Neurol.* 1970;12:101-104.

36.Shapiro SR, Lebowitz R, Colodny AH. Fate of 90 children with ileal conduit urinary diversion a decade later: analysis of complications, pyelography, renal function, and bacteriology. *J Urol.* 1975;114:289-295.

37.Middleton AW, Hendren WH. Ileal conduits in children at the Massachusetts General Hospital from 1955 to 1970. *J Urol.* 1976;118:957.

38.Rickwood AMK, Thomas DG. The upper renal tracts in adolescents and young adults with myelomeningocele. *Z Kinderchir.* 1984;39(suppl II):104-106.

39.Kyker J, Gregory JG, Shah J, Scoenberg HW. Comparison of intermittent catheterization and supravesical diversion in children with meningomyelocele. *J Urol.* 1977;118:90-91.

40.Muralikrishna GS, Rodger RSC, Macdougall AI, Boulton-Jones JM, Allison MEM, Kyle KF, Junor BJR, et al. Renal replacement treatment in patients with spina bifida or spinal cord injury. *Br Med J.* 1989;299:1506.

41.Dorner S. The relationship of physical handicap to stress in families with an adolescent with spina bifida. *Develop Med Child Neurol.* 1975;17:765-776.

42.Lonton AP, O'Sullivan AM, Loughlin AM. Spina bifida adults. *Z Kinderchir.* 1983;38(suppl II):110-112.

43.Blum RW, et al. Ibid.

44.McAndrew I. Adolescents and young people with spina bifida. *Develop Med Child Neurol.* 1979;21:619-629.

45.Castree BJ, Walker JH. The young adult with spina bifida. *Br Med J.* 1981;283:1040-1042.

46.Castaneda AR, Trusler GA, Paul MJ, Blackstone EH, Kirklin JW, Congenital Heart Surgeons Society. The early results of treatment of simple transposition in the current era. *J Thorac Cardiovasc Surg.* 1988;95:14-28.

47.Tew B, et al. Ibid.

48.Smith AD. Adult spina bifida survey in Scotland: Educational attainment and employment. *Z Kinderchir.* 1983;38(suppl II):107-109.

49.Lonton AP, Loughlin AM, O'Sullivan AM. The employment of adults with spina bifida. *Z Kinderchir.* 1984;39(suppl II):132-134.

50.Friedman WF. Congenital heart disease in infancy and childhood. In: Braunwald E, ed. *Heart Disease: A Textbook of Cardiovascular Medicine.* Philadelphia, Pennsylvania: WB Saunders; 1988:896-975.

51.Calder L, Van Praagh R, Van Praagh S, Sears WP, Corwin R, Levy A, et al. Truncus arteriosus communis: clinical, angiocardiographic, and pathologic findings in 100 patients. *Am Heart J.* 1976;92:23-38.

52.Oldham HN Jr, Kakos GS, Jarmakani MM, Sabiston DC Jr. Pulmonary artery banding in infants with complex congenital heart defects. *Ann Thorac Surg.* 1972;13:342.

53.Di Donato RM, Fyfe DA, Puga FJ, Danielson GK, Ritter DG, Edwards WD, et al. Fifteen-year experience with surgical repair of truncus arteriosus. *J Thorac Cardiovasc Surg.* 1985;89:414-422.

54.Marcelletti C, McGoon DC, Danielson GK, Wallace RB, Mair DD. Early and late results of surgical repair of truncus arteriosus. *Circulation.* 1977;55:636-641.

55.Ebert PA, Turley K, Stanger P, Hoffman JIE, Heymann MA, Rudolph AM. Surgical treatment of truncus arteriosus in the first 6 months of life. *Ann Surg.* 1984;200:451-456.

56.Bove EL, Beekman RH, Snider AR, Callow LB, Underhill DJ, Rocchini AP, et al. Repair of truncus arteriosus in the neonate and young infant. *Ann Thorac Surg.* 1989;47:499-506.

57.Boyce SW, Turley K, Yee ES, Verrier ED, Ebert PA. The fate of the 12 mm porcine valved conduit from the right ventricle to the pulmonary artery. *J Thorac Cardiovasc Surg.* 1988;95:201-207.

58.McGoon DC, Danielson GK, Puga FJ, Ritter DG, Mair DD, Ilstrup DM. Late results after extracardiac conduit repair for congenital cardiac defects. *Am J Cardiol.* 1982;49:1741-1749.

59.Jonas RA, Freed MD, Mayer JE, Castaneda AR. Long-term follow-up of patients with synthetic right heart conduits. *Circulation.* 1985;72(suppl II):II-77 - II-83.

60.Kirklin JW. The surgical repair for complete transposition. *Cardiol Young.* 1991;1:13-25.

61.Rashkind WJ, Miller WW. Creation of an atrial septal defect without thoracotomy: a palliative approach to complete transposition of the great arteries. *JAMA.* 1966;196:991-992.

62.Tynan M. Survival of infants with transposition of the great arteries after balloon atrial septostomy. *Lancet.* 1971;1:621-623.

63.Clarkson PM, Barratt-Boyes BG, Neutze JM, Lowe JB. Results over a 10-year period of palliation followed by corrective surgery for complete transposition of the great arteries. *Circulation.* 1972;45:1251-1258.

64.Jonas RA, Sanders SP, Colan SD, Parness IA, Wernovsky G, Nadal-Ginard B, et al. Rapid two-stage arterial switch for TGA and intact septum beyond the neonatal period. *Circulation.* 1988;78(suppl II):II86. Abstract.

65.Quacgcbcur JM, Rohmer J, Ottenkamp J, Buis T, Kirklin JW, Blackstone EH, Brom AG. The arterial switch operation: An eight-year experience. *J Thorac Cardiovasc Surg.* 1986;92:361-384.

66.Wernovsky G, Hougen TJ, Walsh EP, Sholler GF, Colan SD, Sanders SP, et al. Midterm results after the arterial switch operation for transposition of the great arteries with intact ventricular septum: clinical, hemodynamic, echocardiographic, and electrophysiologic data. *Circulation.* 1988;77:1333-1344.

67.Castaneda AR, et al. Ibid.

68.Hayes CJ, Gersony WM. Arrhythmias after the Mustard operation for transposition of the great arteries: a long-term study. *J Am Coll Cardiol.* 1986;7:133-137.

69.Ashraf MH, Cotroneo J, DiMarco D, Subramanian S. Fate of long-term survivors of Mustard procedure (inflow repair) for simple and complex transposition of the great arteries. *Ann Thorac Surg.* 1986;42:385-389.

70.Deanfield J, Camm J, Macartney F, Cartwright T, Douglas J, Drew J, et al. Arrhythmia and late mortality after Mustard and Senning operation for transposition of the great arteries: an eight-year prospective study. *J Thorac Cardiovasc Surg.* 1988;96:569-576.

71.Merrill WH, Stewart JR, Hammon JW, Johns JA, Bender HW Jr. The Senning operation for complete transposition: mid-term physiologic, electrophysiologic, and functional results. *Cardiol Young.* 1991;1:80-83.

72.Duster MC, Bink-Boelkens MTE, Wampler D, Gillette PC, McNamara DG, Cooley DA. Long-term follow-up of dysrhythmias following the Mustard procedure. *Am Heart J.* 1985;109:1323-1326.

73.Turina M, Siebenmann R, Nussbaumer P, Senning A. Long-term outlook after atrial correction of transposition of the great arteries: Cautious optimism. *J Thorac Cardiovasc Surg.* 1988;95:828-835.

74.Flinn CJ, Wolfe GS, Dick M, Campbell RM, Borkat G, Casta A, et al. Cardiac rhythm after the Mustard operation for complete TGA. *New Engl J Med.* 1984;310:1635-1638.

75.Morris CD, Menashe VD. 25-year mortality after surgical repair of congenital heart defect in childhood: a population-based cohort study. *JAMA.* 1991;266:3447-3452.

76.Piccoli G, Pacifico AD, Kirklin JW, Blackstone EH, Kirklin JK, Bargeron LM Jr. Changing results and concepts in the surgical treatment of double-outlet right ventricle: analysis of 137 operations in 126 patients. *Am J Cardiol.* 1983;52:549-554.

77.Sondheimer HM, Freedom RM, Olley PM. Double outlet right ventricle: clinical spectrum and prognosis. *Am J Cardiol.* 1977;39:709.

78.Judson JP, Danielson GK, Puga FJ, Mair DD, McGoon DC. Double-outlet right ventricle: surgical results, 1970-1980. *J Thorac Cardiovasc Surg.* 1983;85:32-40.

79.Shen WK, Holmes DR Jr, Porter CJ, McGoon DC, Ilstrup DM. Sudden death after repair of double-outlet right ventricle. *Circulation.* 1990;81:128-136.

80.Moodie DS, Ritter DG, Tajik AJ, O'Fallon WM. Long-term follow-up in the unoperated univentricular heart. *Am J Cardiol.* 1984;53:1124-1128.

81.Moodie DS, Ritter DG, Tajik AH, McGoon DC, Danielson GK, O'Fallon WM. Long-term follow-up after palliative operation for univentricular heart. *Am J Cardiol.* 1984;53:1648-1651.

82.Bartmus DA, Driscoll DJ, Offord KP, Humes RA, Mair DD, Schaff HV, et al. The modified Fontan operation for children less than 4 years old. *J Am Coll Cardiol.* 1990;15:429-435.

83.Driscoll DJ, Offord KP, Feldt RH, Schaff HV, Puga FJ, Danielson GK. Five- to fifteen-year follow-up after Fontan operation. *Circulation.* 1992;85:469-496.

84.Fontan F, Kirklin JW, Fernandez G, Costa F, Naftel DC, Tritto F, et al. Outcome after a "perfect" Fontan operation. *Circulation.* 1990;81:1520-1536.

85.Stefanelli G, Kirklin JW, Naftel DC, Blackstone EH, Pacifico AD, Kirklin JK, et al. Early and intermediate-term (10-year) results of surgery for univentricular atrioventricular connection ("single ventricle"). *Am J Cardiol.* 1984;54:811-821.

86.Fernandez G, Costa F, Fontan F, Naftel DC, Blackstone EH, Kirklin JW. Prevalence of reoperation for pathway obstruction after Fontan operation. *Ann Thorac Surg.* 1989;48:654-659.

87.Fontan F, Fernandez G, Costa F, Naftel DC, Tritto F, Blackstone EH, et al. The size of the pulmonary arteries and the results of the Fontan operation. *J Thorac Cardiovasc Surg.* 1989;98:711-724.

88.Humes RA, Porter CJ, Mair DD, Rice MJ, Offord KP, Puga FJ, et al. Intermediate follow-up and predicted survival after the modified Fontan procedure for tricuspid atresia and double-inlet ventricle. *Circulation.* 1987;76(suppl III):III-67.

89.Feldt RH, Mair DD, Danielson GK, Wallace RB, McGoon DC. Current status of the septation procedure for univentricular heart. *J Thorac Cardiovasc Surg.* 1981;82:93-97.

90.Pinsky WW, Arciniegas E. Tetralogy of Fallot. *Pediatr Clin N Amer.* 1990;37:179-192.

91.Touati GD, Vouhe PR, Amodeo A, Pouard P, Mauriat P, Leca F, et al. Primary repair of tetralogy of Fallot in infancy. *J Thorac Cardiovasc Surg.* 1990;99:396-403.

92.Walsh EP, Rockenmacher S, Keane JF, Hougen TJ, Lock JE, Castaneda AR. Late results in patients with tetralogy of Fallot repaired during infancy. *Circulation.* 1988;77:1062-1067.

93.Khoury MJ, Cordero JF, Mulinare J, Opitz JM. Selected midline defect associations: a population study. *Pediatrics.* 1989;84:266-272.

94.Zhao HX, Miller DC, Reitz BA, Shumway NE. Surgical repair of tetralogy of Fallot: long-term follow-up with particular emphasis on late death and reoperation. *J Thorac Cardiovasc Surg.* 1985;89:204-220.

95.Haneda K, Togo T, Tabayashi K, Tsuru Y, Mohri H. Long-term results after repair of tetralogy of Fallot. *Tohoku J Exp Med.* 1990;161:319-327.

96.Rosenthal A, Behrendt D, Sloan H, Ferguson P, Snedecor SM, Schork MA. Long-term prognosis (15 to 26 years) after repair of tetralogy of Fallot: I. survival and symptomatic status. *Ann Thorac Surg.* 1984;38:151-156.

97.Horneffer PJ, Zahka KG, Rowe SA, Manolio TA, Gott VL, Reitz BA, et al. Long-term results of total repair of tetralogy of Fallot in childhood. *Ann Thorac Surg.* 1990;50:179-185.

98.Fraser FC. The genetics of cleft lip and cleft palate. *Am J Human Genet.* 1970;22:336-352.

99.Shprintzen RJ, Siegel-Sadewitz VL, Amato J, Goldberg RB. Anomalies associated with cleft lip, cleft palate, or both. *Am J Med Genet.* 1985;20:585-595.

100.Khoury MJ, et al. Ibid.

101.Jones MC. Etiology of facial clefts: prospective evaluation of 428 patients. *Cleft Palate J.* 1988;25:16-20.

102.Rollnick BR, Pruzansky S. Genetic services at a center for craniofacial anomalies. *Cleft Palate J.* 1981;18:304-313.

103.Wyse RKH, Mars M, Al-Mahdawi S, Russell-Eggitt IM, Blake KD. Congenital heart anomalies in patients with clefts of the lip and/or palate. *Cleft Palate J.* 1990;27:258-265.

104.David TJ, Illingworth CA. Diaphragmatic hernia in the southwest of England. *J Med Genet.* 1976;13:253.

105.Hardin MA, Van Demark DR, Morris HL. Long-term speech results of cleft palate speakers with marginal velopharyngeal competence. *J Commun Disord.* 1990;23:401-416.

106.Enemark H, Bolund S, Jorgenson I. Evaluation of unilateral cleft lip and palate treatment: long-term results. *Cleft Palate J.* 1990;27:354-361.

107.Richman LC, Eliason MJ, Lindgren SD. Reading disability in children with clefts. *Cleft Palate J.* 1988;25:21-25.

108.McWilliams BJ, Paradise LP. Educational, occupational, and marital status of cleft palate adults. *Cleft Palate J.* 1973;10:223-229.

109.Peter JP, Chinsky RR, Fisher MJ. Sociological aspects of cleft palate adults. IV. social integration. *Cleft Palate J.* 1975;12:304-310.

110.Manning PB, Morgan RA, Coran AG, Wesley JR, Polley TZ, Behrendt DM, et al. Fifty years' experience with esophageal atresia and tracheoesophageal fistula. *Ann Surg.* 1986;204:446-453.

111.Louhimo I, Lindahl H. Esophageal atresia: primary results of 500 consecutively treated patients. *J Pediatr Surg.* 1983;18:217-229.

112.Beasley SW, Shann FA, Myers NA, Auldist AW. Developments in the management of oesophageal atresia and tracheoesophageal fistulas. *Med J Austr.* 1989;150:501-503.

121.Martinez-Frias ML, Frias JL, Salvador J. Clinical/epidemiological analysis of malformations. *Am J Med Genetics.* 1989;35:121-125.

114.Fraser C, Baird PA, Sadovnick AD. A comparison of incidence trends for esophageal atresia and tracheoesophageal fistula, and infectious disease. *Teratology.* 1987;36:363-369.

115.Ein SH, Shandling B, Wesson D, Filler RM. Esophageal atresia with distal tracheoesophageal fistula: associated anomalies and prognosis in the 1980's. *J Pediatr Surg.* 1989;24:1055-1059.

116.Holder TM, Ashcraft KW, Sharp RJ, Amoury RA. Care of infants with esophageal atresia, tracheoesophageal fistula, and associated anomalies. *J Thorac Cardiovasc Surg.* 1987;94:828-835.

117.Bishop PJ, Klein MD, Philippart AI, Hixson DS, Hertzler JH. Transpleural repair of esophageal atresia without a primary gastrostomy: 240 patients treated between 1951 and 1983. *J Pediatr Surg.* 1985;20:823-828.

118.Shaul DB, Schwartz MZ, Marr CC, Tyson KRT. Primary repair without routine gastrostomy is the treatment of choice for neonates with esophageal atresia and tracheoesophageal fistula. *Arch Surg.* 1989;124:1188-1191.

119.Spitz L, Kiely E, Brereton RJ. Esophageal atresia: Five year experience with 148 cases. *J Pediatr Surg.* 1987;22:103-108.

120.McKinnon LJ, Kosloske AM. Prediction and prevention of anastomotic complications of esophageal atresia and tracheoesophageal fistula. *J Pediatr Surg.* 1990;25:778-781.

121.Chittmittrapap S, Spitz L, Kiely EM, Brereton RJ. Anastomotic stricture following repair of esophageal atresia. *J Pediatr Surg.* 1990;25:508-511.

122.Dudley NE, Phelan PD. Respiratory complications of long-term survivors of oesophageal atresia. *Arch Dis Childhood.* 1976;51:279-282.

123.Biller JA, Allen JL, Schuster SR, Treves ST, Winter HS. Long-term evaluation of esophageal and pulmonary function in patients with repaired esophageal atresia and tracheoesophageal fistula. *Digest Dis Sci.* 1987;32:985-990.

124.David TJ, Illingworth CA. Ibid.

125.Osebold WR, Soper RT. Congenital posterolateral diaphragmatic hernia past infancy. *Am J Surg.* 1976;131:748-754.

126.Gregory GA, Kitterman JA. Lesions of the diaphragm. In: Rudolph AM, Hoffman JIE, Randolph CD, eds. *Rudolph's Pediatrics.* Norwalk, Connecticut: Appleton Lange; 1991:1474-1478.

127.Siebert JR, Benjamin DR. Chest size and symmetry in congenital diaphragmatic hernia. *J Pediatr Surg.* 1987;22:394-396.

128.Siebert JR, Haas JE, Beckwith JB. Left ventricular hypoplasia and congenital diaphragmatic hernia. *J Pediatr Surg.* 1984;19:567-571.

129.Adelman S, Benson CD. Bochdalek hernias in infants: factors determining mortality. *J Pediatr Surg.* 1976;11:569-573.

130.Benjamin DR, Juul S, Siebert JR. Congenital posterolateral diaphragmatic hernia: associated malformations. *J Pediatr Surg.* 1988;23:899-903.

131.Harrison MR, de Lorimier AA. Congenital diaphragmatic hernia. *Surg Clin N Amer.* 1981;61:1023-1035.

132.Bohn D, Tamura M, Perrin D, Barker G, Rabinovitch M. Ventilatory predictors of pulmonary hypoplasia in congenital diaphragmatic hernia, confirmed by morphologic assessment. *J Pediatr.* 1987;111:423-431.

133.Heiss K, Manning P, Oldham KT, Coran AG, Polley TZ, Wesley JR, et al. Reversal of mortality for congenital diaphragmatic hernia with ECMO. *Ann Surg.* 1989;209:225-230.

134.Weber TR, Connors RH, Pennington DG, Westfall S, Keenan W, Kotagal S, et al. Neonatal diaphragmatic hernia: an improving outlook with extracorporeal membrane oxygenation. *Arch Surg.* 1987;122:615-618.

135.Van Meurs KP, Newman KD, Anderson KD, Short BL. Effect of extracorporeal membrane oxygenation on survival of infants with congenital diaphragmatic hernia. *J Pediatr.* 1990;117:954-960.

136.Freyschuss U, Lannergren K, Frenckner B. Lung function after repair of congenital diaphragmatic hernia. *Acta Pediatr Scan.* 1984;73:589-593.

137.Reid IS, Hutcherson RJ. Long-term follow-up of patients with congenital diaphragmatic hernia. *J Pediatr Surg.* 1976;11:939-942.

138.Falconer AR, Brown RA, Helms P, Gordon I, Baron JA. Pulmonary sequelae in survivors of congenital diaphragmatic hernia. *Thorax.* 1990;45:126-129.

139.Stolar CJH, Levy JP, Dillon PW, Reyes C, Belamarich P, Berdon WE. Anatomic and functional abnormalities of the esophagus in infants surviving congenital diaphragmatic hernia. *Am J Surg.* 1990;159:204-207.

140.Miller RC. Complicated intestinal atresias. *Ann Surg.* 1979;189:607-611.

141.Rescorla FJ, Grosfeld JL. Intestinal atresia and stenosis: analysis of survival in 120 cases. *Surgery.* 1985;98:668-676.

142.Weber TR, Lewis JE, Mooney D, Connors R. Duodenal atresia: a comparison of techniques of repair. *J Pediatr Surg.* 1986;21:1133-1136.

143.Harberg FJ, Pokorny WJ, Hahn H. Congenital duodenal obstruction: a review of 65 cases. *Am J Surg.* 1979;138:825-828.

144.Kimura K, Mukohara N, Nishijima E, Muraji T, Tsugawa C, Matsumoto Y. Diamond-shaped anastomosis for duodenal atresia: an experience with 44 patients over 15 years. *J Pediatr Surg.* 1990;25:977-979.

145.Spigland N, Yazbeck S. Complications associated with surgical treatment of congenital intrinsic duodenal obstruction. *J Pediatr Surg.* 1990;25:1127-1130.

146.Paterson-Brown S, Stalewski H, Brereton RJ. Neonatal small bowel atresia, stenosis, and segmental dilatation. *Br J Surg.* 1991;78:83-86.

147.Smith GHH, Glasson M. Intestinal atresia: factors affecting survival. *Aust NZ J Surg.* 1989;59:151-156.

148.Manning C, Strauss A, Gyepes MT. Jejunal atresia with "apple peel" deformity: a report of eight survivors. *J Perinatol.* 1989;9:281-286.

149.Danismend EN, Frank JD, Brown S. Morbidity and mortality in small bowel atresia: jejuno-ileal atresia. *Z Kinderchir.* 1987;42:17-18.

150.Powell RW, Raffensperger JG. Congenital colonic atresia. *J Pediatr Surg.* 1982; 17:166-170.

151.Pohlson EC, Hatch EI, Glick PL, Tapper D. Individualized management of colonic atresia. *Am J Surg.* 1988;155:690-692.

152.Thorner PS,

153.Stephens FD, Smith ED. *Classification, identification, and assessment of surgical treatment of anorectal anomalies.* Racine, Wisconsin: Report of Wingspread Workshop; 1980.

154.Kiesewetter WB, Hoon A. Imperforate anus: an analysis of mortalities during a 25-year period. *Progress Pediatr Surg.* 1979;13:211-220.

155.Kiesewetter WB, Chang JHT. Imperforate anus: a five to thirty year follow-up perspective. *Progress Pediatr Surg.* 1977;10:111-120.

156.Holschneider AM. Treatment and functional results of anorectal continence in children with imperforate anus. *Acta Chir Belg.* 1983;83:191-204.

157.Fleming SE, Hall R, Gysler M, McLorie GA. Imperforate anus in females: frequency of genital tract involvement, incidence of associated anomalies, and functional outcome. *J Pediatr Surg.* 1986;21:146-150.

158.Scharli AF, Holschneider AM, Kraeft H, Illi O. Causes of postoperative mortality in anorectal malformations: analysis and conclusions regarding therapy. *Progress Pediatr Surg.* 1977;10:225-230.

159.Khoury MJ, Cordero JF, Greenberg F, et al. A population study of the VACTERL association. *Pediatrics.* 1983;71:815.

160.Noe HN, Marshall JH, Edwards OP. Nodular renal blastema in the multicystic kidney. *J Urol.* 1989; 142:486-488.

161.Pedicelli G, Jequier S, Bowen A, Boisvert J. Multicystic dysplastic kidneys: spontaneous regression demonstrated with US. *Radiology.* 1986;160:23.

162.Hashimoto BE, Filly RA, Callen PW. Multicystic dysplastic kidney in utero: changing appearnace on US. *Radiology.* 1986;159:107.

163.Avni EF, Thoua Y, Lalmand B, et al. Multicystic dysplastic kidney: natural history from in utero diagnosis and postnatal followup. *J Urol.* 1987; 138:1420.

164.Nixon HH, Puri P. The results of treatment of anorectal anomalies: a thirteen to twenty year follow-up. *J Pediatr Surg.* 1977;12:27-37.

165.Iwai N, Yanagihara J, Tokiwa K, Degiuchi E, Takahashi T. Results of surgical correction of anorectal malformations: a 10-30 year follow-up. *Ann Surg.* 1988;207:219-222.

166.Pedicelli G, et al. Ibid.

167.Templeton JM, Ditesheim JA. High imperforate anus: quantitative results of long-term fecal continence. *J Pediatr Surg.* 1985;20:645-652.

168.Ong NT, Beasley SW. Long-term continence in patients with high and intermediate anorectal anomalies treated by sacroperineal (Stephens) rectoplasty. *J Pediatr Surg.* 1991;26:44-48.

169.Potter EL. Bilateral renal agenesis. *J Pediatr.* 1946;29:68.

170.Thomas IT, Smith DW. Oligohydramnios, cause of the nonrenal features of Potter's syndrome, including pulmonary hypoplasia. *J Pediatr.* 1974;84:811-814.

171.Thorner PS, Arbus GS, Celermajer DS, Baumal R. Focal segmental glomerulosclerosis and progressive renal failure associated with a unilateral kidney. *Pediatrics.* 1984;73:806.

172.Gutierrez-Millet V, Nieto J, Praga M, et al. Focal glomerulosclerosis and proteinuria in patients with solitary kidneys. *Arch Intern Med.* 1986;146:705.

173.Emanuel B, Nachman R, Aronson L, et al. Congenital solitary kidney. *Am J Dis Child.* 1974;127:17.

174.Zilleruelo G, Freundlich M, Abitbol C, Dominguez N, Montane B, Strauss J. *Natural history of congenital anomalies of the kidney and urinary tract.*

175.Cendron J, Gubler JP, Valayer J, Kiriakos S. Dysplasie multicystique du rein chez l' enfant. *J d'Urol Nephrol.* 1973;79:773.

176.Bloom DA, Brosman S. The multicystic kidney. *J Urol.* 1978;120:211-215.

177.Glick PL, Harrison MR, Noall R, et al. Correction of congenital hydronephrosis in utero. III. early mid-trimester urethral obstruction produces renal dysplasia. *J Pediatr Surg.* 1983;18:681-687.

178.Glick PL, Harrison MR, Adzick NS, et al. Correction of congenital hydronephrosis in utero. IV. in utero decompression prevents renal dysplasia. *J Pediatr Surg.* 1984;19:649-657.

179.Gordon AC, Thomas DFM, Arthur RJ, Irving HC. Multicystic dysplastic kidney: is nephrectomy still appropriate? *J Urol.* 1988;140:1231-1234.

180.Vinocur L, Slovis TL, Perlmutter AD, Watts FB, Chang CH. Follow-up studies of multicystic dysplastic kidneys. *Radiology.* 1988;167:311-315.

181.Barrett DM, Wineland RE. Renal cell carcinoma in multicystic dysplastic kidney. *Urology.* 1980;15:152.

182.Birken G, King D, Vane D, Lloyd T. Renal cell carcinoma arising in a multicystic dysplastic kidney. *J Pediatr Surg.* 1985;20:619.

183.Dimmick JE, Johnson HW, Coleman GU, Carter M. Wilms tumorlet, nodular renal blastema and multicystic renal dysplasia. *J Urol.* 1989;142:484.

184.Noe HN, Marshall JH, Edwards OP. Nodular renal blastema in the multicystic kidney. *J Urol.* 1989;142:486-488.

185.Pedicelli G, Jequier S, Bowen A, Boisvert J. Multicystic dysplastic kidneys: spontaneous regression demonstrated with US. *Radiology.* 1986;160:23.

186.Hashimoto BE, Filly RA, Callen PW. Multicystic dysplastic kidney in utero: changing appearance on US. *Radiology.* 1986;159:107.

187.Avni EF, Thoua Y, Lalmand B, et al. Multicystic dysplastic kidney: natural history from in utero diagnosis and postnatal followup. *J Urol.* 1987;138:1420.

188.Chen YH, Stapleton FB, Roy S III, Noe HN. Neonatal hypertension from a unilateral multicystic, dysplastic kidney. *J Urol.* 1985;133:664.

189.Brown T, Mandell J, Lebowitz RL. Neonatal hydronephrosis in the era of sonography. *AJR*. 1987;148:959-963.

190.Steele BT, De Maria J, Toi A, Stafford A, Hunter D, Caco C. Neonatal outcome of fetuses with urinary tract abnormalities diagnosed by prenatal ultrasonography. *CMAJ*. 1987;137:117-120.

191.Bernstein GT, Mandell J, Lebowitz RL, Bauer SB, Colodny AH, Retik AB. Ureteropelvic junction obstruction in the neonate. *J Urol*. 1988;140:1216-1221.

192.Wolpert JJ, Woodard JR, Parrott TS. Pyeloplasty in the young infant. *J Urol*. 1989;142:573-575.

193.Glick PL, Harrison MR, Adzick NS, et al. Management of the fetus with congenital hydronephrosis. II. prognostic criteria and selection for treatment. *J Pediatr Surg*. 1985;20:376-387.

194.Chierici R, Riccipetitoni G, Tamisari L, Vesce F, Zanella B, Merlo L, Vigi V. Conservative management of urinary abnormalities detected in utero. *Fetal Ther*. 1989;4:43-48.

195.Dowling KJ, Harmon EP, Ortenberg J, Polanco E, Evans BB. Ureteropelvic junction obstruction: effect of pyeloplasty on renal function. *J Urol*. 1988;140:1227-1230.

196.King LR, Hatcher PA. Natural history of fetal and neonatal hydronephrosis. *Urology*. 1990;35:443-448.

197.King LR. Evaluation and management of ureteropelvic obstruction in the neonate. In: Gonzales ET, Roth D, eds. *Common problems in pediatric urology*. St. Louis, Missouri: Mosby-Year Book, Inc.; 1991.

198.Ransley PG, Dhillon HK, Gordon I, Duffy PG, Dillon MJ, Barratt TM. The postnatal management of hydronephrosis diagnosed by prenatal ultrasound. *J Urol*. 1990;144:584-587.

199.Guys JM, Borella F, Monfort G. Uteropelvic junction obstruction: prenatal diagnosis and neonatal surgery in 47 cases. *J Pediatr Surg*. 1988;23:156-158.

200.Nguyen DH, Aliabadi H, Ercole CJ, Gonzales R. Nonintubated Anderson-Hynes repair of ureteropelvic junction obstruction in 60 patients. *J Urol*. 1989;142:704-706.

201.Van Cangh PJ, Jorion JL, Wese FX, Opsomer RJ. Endoureteropyelotomy: percutaneous treatment of ureteropelvic junction obstruction. *J Urol*. 1989;141:1317-1322.

234   The Cost of Birth Defects

202.Hollowell JG, Altman HG, McC Snyder H III, Duckett JW. Coexisting ureteropelvic junction obstruction and vesicoureteral reflux: diagnostic and therapeutic implications. *J Urol.* 1989;142:490-493.

203.Keating MA, Escala J, McC Snyder III, Heyman S, Duckett JW. Changing concepts in management of primary obstructive megaureter. *J Urol.* 1989;142:636-640.

204.Peters CA, Mandell J, Lebowitz RL, Colodny AH, Bauer SB, Hendren WH, et al. Congenital obstructed megaureters in early infancy: diagnosis and treatment. *J Urol.* 1989;142:641-645.

205.Kalicinski ZH, Kansy K, Kotarbinska B, et al. Surgery of megaureters: modification of Hendren's operation. *J Pediatr Surg.* 1977;12:183.

206.Warshaw BL, Edelbrock HH, Ettenger RB, et al. Progression to end-stage renal disease in children with obstructive uropathy. *J Pediatr.* 1982;100:183.

207.Frantz CH, O'Rahilly R. Congenital skeletal limb deficiencies. *J Bone Joint Surg.* 1961;43-A:1202-1224.

208.Burtch RL. Classification nomenclature for congenital skeletal limb deficiencies. In: Kekikian H, ed. *Congenital Deformities of the Hand and Forearm.* Philadelphia, Pennsulvania: WB Saunders Co.; 1974.

209.Swanson AB. Congenital limb defects: classification and treatment. *Clinical Symposia.* 1981;33(3):3-32.

210.Froster-Iskenius UG, Baird PA. Limb reduction defects in over one million consecutive livebirths. *Teratology.* 1989;39:127-135.

211.Cheng JCY, Chow SK, Leung PC. Classification of 578 cases of congenital upper limb anomalies with the IFSSH system-a 10 years' experience. *J Hand Surg.* 1987;12A:1055-1060.

212.Leung PC, Chan KM, Cheng JCY. Congenital anomalies of the upper limb among the Chinese population in Hong Kong. *J Hand Surg.* 1982;7:563-565.

213.Lamb DW, Wynne-Davies R, Soto L. An estimate of the population frequency of congenital malformations of the upper limb. *J Hand Surg.* 1982;7:557-562.

214.Martinez-Frias ML, Frias JL, Salvador J. Clinical/epidemiological analysis of malformations. *Am J Med Genet.* 1989;35:121-125.

215.Kallen B, Rahmani TMZ, Winberg J. Infants with congenital limb reduction registered in the Swedish Register of Congenital Malformations. *Teratology.* 1984;29:73-85.

216.Jones KL. *Smith's Recognizable Patterns of Human Malformation.* 4th ed. Philadelphia: WB Saunders Co.; 1988.

217.Froster-Iskenius UG, Baird PA. Amelia: incidence and associated defects in a large population. *Teratology.* 1990;41:23-31.

218.Mason KJ. Congenital orthopedic anomalies and their impact on the family. *Nursing Clin North Am.* 1991;26:1-19.

219.Ashley RK, Vallier GT, Skinner SR. Gait analysis in pediatric lower extremity amputees. *Orthop Rev.* 1992;21:745-749.

220.Achterman C, Kalamchi A. Congenital deficiency of the fibula. *J Bone Joint Surg.* 1979;61-B:133-137.

221.Hootnick D, Boyd NA, Fixsen JA, Lloyd-Roberts GC. The natural history and management of congenital short tibia with dysplasia or absence of the fibula: a preliminary report. *J Bone Joint Surg.* 1977;59-B:267-271.

222.Thomas IH, Williams PF. The Gruca operation for congenital absence of the fibula. *J Bone Joint Surg.* 1987;69-B:587-592.

223.Aitken GT. Amputation as a treatment for certain lower-extremity congenital abnormalities. *J Bone Joint Surg.* 1959;41-A:1267-1285.

224.Wood WL, Zlotsky N, Westin GW. Congenital absence of the fibula: treatment by Syme amputation-Indications and techniques. *J Bone Joint Surg.* 1965;47-A:1159-1169.

225.Mazct R. Syme's amputation: a follow-up study of fifty-one adults and thirty-two children. *J Bone Joint Surg.* 1968;50-A:1549-1563.

226.Westin GW, Sakai DN, Wood WL. Congenital longitudinal deficiency of the fibula: follow-up of treatment by Syme amputation. *J Bone Joint Surg.* 1976;58-A:492-496.

227.Kalamchi A, Dawe RV. Congenital deficiency of the tibia. *J Bone Joint Surg.* 1985;67-B:581-584.

228.Jones D, Barnes J, Lloyd-Roberts GC. Congenital aplasia and dysplasia of the tibia with intact fibula: classification and management. *J Bone Joint Surg.* 1978;60-B:31-39.

229.Brown FW, Pohnert WH. Construction of a knee joint in meromelia tibia (congenital absence of the tibia): a 15 year follow-up study. *J Bone Joint Surg.* 54-A:1333.

230.Loder RT, Herring JA. Fibular transfer for congenital absence of the tibia: a reassessment. *J Pediatr Orthop.* 1987;7:8-13.

231.Schoenecker PL, Capelli AM, Millar EA, Sheen MR, Haher T, Aiona MD, et al. Congenital longitudinal deficiency of the tibia. *J Bone Joint Surg.* 1989;71-A:278-287.

232.Epps CH, Schneider PL. Treatment of hemimelias of the lower extremity: long-term results. *J Bone Joint Surg.* 1989;71-A:273-277.

233.Gillespie R, Torode IP. Classification and management of congenital abnormalities of the femur. *J Bone Joint Surg.* 1983;65-B:557-568.

234.Pappas AM. Congenital abnormalities of the femur and related lower extremity malformations: classification and treatment. *J Pediatr Orthop.* 1983;3:45-60.

235.Kritter AE. Tibial rotation-plasty for proximal femoral focal deficiency. *J Bone Joint Surg.* 1977;59-A:927-933.

236.Lidge RT. The treatment of congenital radial deficient clubhand–a technique. *J Bone Joint Surg.* 1957;39-A:687.

237.Swanson AB. The Krukenberg procedure in the juvenile amputee. *J Bone Joint Surg.* 1964;46-A:1540-1548.

238.de Vries PA. The pathogenesis of gastroschisis and omphalocele. *J Pediatr Surg.* 1980;15:245-251.

239.Torfs C, Curry C, Roeper P. Gastroschisis. *J Pediatr.* 1990;116:1-6.

240.Tibboel D, Vermey-Keers C, Kluck P, et al. The natural history of gastroschisis during fetal life: development of the fibrous coating on the bowel loops. *Teratology.* 1986;33:267.

241.van Geijn EJ, van Vugt JM, Sollie JE, van Geijn HP. Ultrasonographic diagnosis and perinatal management of fetal abdominal wall defects. *Fetal Diag Ther.* 1991;6:2-10.

242.Gilbert WM, Nicolaides KH. Fetal omphalocele: associated malformations and chromosomal defects. *Obstetr Gynecol.* 1987;70:633-635.

243.Grosfeld JL, Weber TR. Congenital abdominal wall defects: gastroschisis and omphalocele. *Current Problems in Surg.* 1982;158-213.

244.Greenwood RD, Rosenthal A, Nadas AS. Cardiovascular malformations associated with omphaloceles. *J Pediatr.* 1974;85:818.

245.Lindham S. Omphalocele and gastroschisis in Sweden 1965-1976. *Acta Pediatr Scand.* 1981;70:55-60.

246.Roeper PJ, Harris J, Lee G, Neutra R. Secular rates and correlates for gastroschisis in California (1968-1977). *Teratology.* 1987;35:203-210.

247.Martinez-Frias ML, Salvador J, Prieto L, Zaplana J. Epidemiological study of gastroschisis and omphalocele in Spain. *Teratology.* 1984;29:377-382.

248.Mabogunje OA, Mahour GH. Omphalocele and gastroschisis: trends in survival across two decades. *Am J Surg.* 1984;148:679-686.

249.Yazbeck S, Ndoye M, Khan AH. Omphalocele: a 25-year experience. *J Pediatr Surg.* 1986;21:761-763.

250.Tucci M, Bard H. The associated anomalies that determine prognosis in congenital omphaloceles. *Am J Obstet Gynecol.* 1990;163:1646-1649.

251.Lenke RR, Hatch JR, Edwin I. Fetal gastroschisis: a preliminary report advocating the use of cesarean section. *Obstet Gynecol.* 1986;67:395-398.

252.Fitzsimmons J, Nyberg DA, Cyr DR, Hatch E. Perinatal management of gastroschisis. *Obstet Gynecol.* 1988;71:910-913.

253.Lewis DF, Towers CV, Garite TJ, Jackson DN, Nageotte MP, Major CA. Fetal gastroschisis and omphalocele: is cesarean section the best mode of delivery? *Am J Obstet Gynecol.* 1990;163:773-775.

254.Sermer M, Benzie RJ, Pitson L, Carr M, Skidmore M. Prenatal diagnosis and management of congenital defects of the anterior abdominal wall. *Am J Obstet Gynecol.* 1987;156:308-312.

255.Moretti M, Khouri A, Rodriguez J, Lobe T, Shaver D, Sibai B. The effect of mode of delivery on the perinatal outcome in fetuses with abdominal wall defects. *Am J Obstet Gynecol.* 1990;163:833-838.

256.Sipes SL, Weiner CP, Sipes DR 2nd, Grant SS, Williamson RA. Gastroschisis and omphalocele: does either antenatal diagnosis or route of delivery make a difference in perinatal outcome? *Obstet Gynecol.* 1990;76:195-199.

257.Meller JL, Reyes HM, Loeff DS. Gastroschisis and omphalocele. *Clin Perinatol.* 1989;16:113-122.

258.Gongaware RD, Marino BL, Smith RM, Sacks LM, Morrison JV Jr. Management of gastroschisis. *Amer Surgeon.* 1987;53:468-471.

259.Lindham S, Ramel S. A retrospective study of 91 cases with gastroschisis or omphalocele 1956-1985. *Z Kinderchir.* 1987;42:366-370.

260.Lafferty PM, Emmerson AJ, Fleming PJ, Frank JD, Noblett HR. Anterior abdominal wall defects. *Arch Dis Child.* 1989;64:1029-1031.

261.Bryant MS, Tepas JJ, Mollitt DL, Talbert JL, String DL. The effect of initial operative repair on the recovery of intestinal function in gastroschisis. *Amer Surgeon.* 1989;55:209-211.

262.Muraji T, Tsugawa C, Nishijima E, Tanano H, Matsumoto Y, Kimura K. Gastroschisis: a 17-year experience. *J Pediatr Surg.* 1989;24:343-345.

263.Stringer MD, Brereton RJ, Wright VM. Controversies in the management of gastroschisis: a study of 40 patients. *Arch Dis Child.* 1991;66(1 spec no):34-36.

264.Mercer S, Mercer B, D'Alton ME, Soucy P. Gastroschisis: ultrasonographic diagnosis, perinatal embryology, surgical and obstetric treatment and outcomes. *Can J Surg.* 1988;31:25-26.

265.Di Lorenzo M, Yazbeck S, Ducharme JC. Gastroschisis: a 15-year experience. *J Pediatr Surg.* 1987;22:710-712.

266.Oldham KT, Coran AG, Drongowski RA, Baker PJ, Wesley JR, Polley TZ Jr. The development of necrotizing enterocolitis following repair of gastroschisis: a surprisingly high incidence. *J Pediatr Surg.* 1988;23:945-949.

267.Touloukian RJ, Spackman TJ. Gastroschisis: function and radiographic appearance following repair. *J Pediatr Surg.* 1971;6:427.

268.Berseth CL, Malachowski N, Cohn RB, Sunshine P. Longitudinal growth and late morbidity of survivors of gastroschisis and omphalocele. *J Pediatr Gastroenter Nutr.* 1982;1:375-379.

269.Lindham S. Long-term results in children with omphalocele and gastroschisis: a follow-up study. *Z Kinderchir.* 1984;39:164-167.

270.Tarnowski KJ, King DR, Green L, Ginn-Pease ME. Congenital gastrointestinal anomalies: psychosocial functioning of children with imperforate anus, gastroschisis, and omphalocele. *J Consult Clin Psychol.* 1991;59:587-590.

271.Hall B. Mongolism in newborn infants. *Clin Pediatr.* 1966;5:4.

272.Pueschel SM, Rynders JE. *Down Syndrome: Advances in Biomedicine and the Behavioral Sciences.* Cambridge, Massachusetts: Ware Press; 1982.

273.Baird P, Sadovnick A. Life expectancy in Down syndrome. *J Pediatr.* 1987;110:849-854.

274.Fabia J, Drolette M. Life table up to age 10 for mongols with and without congenital heart defect. *J Ment Defic Res.* 1970;14:235-242.

275.Malone Q. Mortality and survival of the Down's syndrome population in Western Australia. *J Ment Defic Res.* 1988;32:59-65.

276.McGrother C, Marshall B. Recent trends in incidence, morbidity and survival in Down's syndrome. *J Ment Defic Res.* 1990;34:49-57.

277.Schneider D, Zahka K, Clark E, Neill C. Patterns of cardiac care in infants with Down syndrome. *AJDC.* 1989;143:363-365.

278.Mathew P, Moodie D, Sterba R, Murphy D, Rosenkranz E, Homa A. Long term follow-up of children with Down syndrome with cardiac lesions. *Clin Pediatr.* 1990;29:569-574.

279.Thase ME. Longevity and mortality in Down's syndrome. *J Ment Defic Res.* 1982;26:177-192.

280.Fabia J, Drolette M. Malformations and leukemia in children with Down's syndrome. *Pediatrics.* 1970;45:60-70.

281.Knox GE, Bensel RW. Gastrointestinal malformations in Down's syndrome. *Minn Med.* 1972;55:542-544.

282.Lowe R. The eyes in mongolism. *Br J Ophthalmol.* 1949;33:131-154.

283.Pueschel SM, Scola FH, Tupper TB, Pezzullo JC. Skeletal anomalies of the upper cervical spine in children with Down syndrome. *J Pediatr Orthop.* 1990;10:607-611.

284.Hook EB, Chambers GM. Estimated rates of Down syndrome in live births by one year maternal age intervals for mothers aged 20-49 in a New York State study–implications of the risk figures for genetic counseling and cost-benefit analysis of prenatal diagnosis programs. *Birth Defects Original Article Series*. 1977;13(3A):123-141.

285.Dykes J. *Ten Thousand Severely Handicapped Children in New South Wales and the Australian Capital Territory*. Canberra: Australian Government Publishing Service; 1978.

286.Eyman RK, Call TL, White JF. Life expectancy of persons with Down syndrome. *Am J Ment Retard*. 1991;95:603-612.

287.Sare Z, Ruvalcaba RHA, Kelley VC. Prevalence of thyroid disorder in Down syndrome. *Clin Genet*. 1978;14:154-158.

288.Friedman DL, Kastner T, Pond WS, O'Brien DR. Thyroid dysfunction in individuals with Down syndrome. *Arch Intern Med*. 1989;149:1990-1993.

289.Dinani S, Carpenter S. Down's syndrome and thyroid disorder. *J Ment Defic Res*. 1990;34:187-193.

290.Pozzan GB, Rigon F, Girelli ME, Rubello D, Busnardo B, Baccichetti C. Thyroid function in patients with Down syndrome: preliminary results from non-institutionalized patients in the Veneto region. *Am J Med Genet*. 1990;7(suppl):57-58.

291.Pueschel SM, Pezzullo JC. Thyroid dysfunction in Down syndrome. *AJDC*. 1985;139:636-639.

292.Mendez AA, Keret D, MacEwen GD. Treatment of patellofemoral instability in Down's syndrome. *Clin Orthop*. 1988;234:148-158.

293.Semine AA, Ertel AN, Goldberg MJ, Bull MJ. Cervical-spine instability in children with Down syndrome (Trisomy 21). *J Bone Joint Surg*. 1978;60-A:649-652.

294.Elliott S, Morton R, Whitelaw R. Atlantoaxial instability and abnormalities of the odontoid in Down's syndrome. *Arch Dis Child*. 1988;63:1484-1489.

295.Pueshcel S, Scola F. Atlantoaxial instability in individuals with Down Syndrome: epidemiologic, radiographic, and clinical studies. *Pediatrics*. 1987;80:555-560.

296.Davidson RG. Atlantoaxial instability in individuals with Down syndrome: a fresh look at the evidence. *Pediatrics*. 1988;81:857-865.

297.Goldhaber SZ, Brown WD, St. John Sutton MG. High frequency of mitral valve prolapse and aortic regurgitation among asymptomatic adults with Down's syndrome. *JAMA.* 1987;258:1793-1795.

298.Barnett ML, Friedman D, Kastner T. The prevalence of mitral valve prolapse in patients with Down's syndrome: implications for dental management. *Oral Surg Oral Med Oral Pathol.* 1988;66:445-447.

299.Davies B. Auditory disorders in Down's syndrome. *Scand Audiol Suppl.* 1988;30:65-68.

300.Balkany TJ, Downs MP, Jafek BW, Krajicek MJ. Hearing loss in Down's syndrome. *Clin Paediatr.* 1979;18(2):116.

301.Brooks DN, Wooley H, Kanjial GC. Hearing loss and middle ear disorders in patients with Down's syndrome. *J Ment Defic Res.* 1972;16:21.

302.Cunningham C, McArthur K. Hearing loss and treatment in young Down's syndrome children. *Child: Care, Health, Dev.* 1981;7:357-374.

303.Catalano R. Down syndrome. *Surv Ophthalmol.* 1990;34:385-398.

304.Walsh S. Keratoconus and blindness in 469 institutionalized subjects with Down syndrome and other causes of mental retardation. *J Ment Defic Res.* 1981;25:243-251.

305.Eissler R, Longenecker LP. The common eye findings in mongolism. *Am J Ophthalmol.* 1962;54:398-406.

306.Gaynon MW, Schimek RA. Down's syndrome: a ten-year group study. *Ann Ophthalmol.* 1977;9:1493-1497.

307.Hiles DA, Hoyme SH, McFarlane F. Down's syndrome and strabismus. *Am Orthop J.* 1974;24:63-68.

308.Shapiro MB, France TD. The ocular features of Down's syndrome. *Am J Ophthalmol.* 1985;99:659-663.

309.Veall RM. The prevalence of epilepsy among mongols related to age. *J Ment Defic Res.* 1974;18:99-105.

310.Moore BC. Some characteristics of institutionalized mongols. *J Ment Defic Res.* 1973;17:46-51.

311.Pueschel SM, Louis S, McKnight P. Seizure disorders in Down syndrome. *Arch Neurol.* 1991;48:318-320.

312.Forsgren L, Edvinsson S, Blomquist H, Heijbel J, Sidenvall R. Epilepsy in a population of mentally retarded children and adults. *Epilepsy Res.* 1990;6:234-248.

313.Romano C, Tine A, Fazio G, Rizzo R, Colognola RM, Sorge G, et al. Seizures in patients with Trisomy 21. *Am J Med Genet Suppl.* 1990;7:298-300.

314.Stafstrom CE, Patxot OF, Gilmore HE, Wisniewski KE. Seizures in children with Down syndrome: Etiology, characteristics and outcome. *Dev Med Child Neurol.* 1991;33:191-200.

315.LeBerre C, Journel H, Lucas J, LeMee F, Betremieux P, Roussey M, LeMarec B. L' epilepsie chez le trisomique 21. *Ann Pediatr (Paris).* 1986;33:579-585.

316.McVicker RW, Shanks OEP, McClelland RJ. Prevalence and associated features of epilepsy in adults with Down syndrome. *Br J Psychiatry.* 1994;164:528-532.

317.Southall DP, Stebbens VA, Mirza R, Lang MH, Croft CB, Shinebourne EA. Upper airway obstruction with hypoxemia and sleep disruption in Down syndrome. *Dev Med Child Neurol.* 1987;29:734-742.

318.Marcus CL, Keens TG, Bautista DB, von Pechmann WS, Ward SLD. Obstructive sleep apnea in children with Down syndrome. *Pediatrics.* 1991;88:132-139.

319.Cutress TW. Periodontal disease and oral hygiene in trisomy 21. *Arch Oral Biol.* 1971;16:1345-1350.

320.Ugazio AG, Maccario R, Notarangelo LD, Burgio GR. Immunology of Down syndrome: a review. *Am J Med Genet Suppl.* 1990;7:204-212.

321.Fong C, Brodeur GM. Down's syndrome and leukemia: epidemiology, genetics, cytogenetics and mechanisms of leukemogenesis. *Cancer Genet Cytogenet.* 1987;28:55-76.

322.Holland WW, Doll R, Carter CO. The mortality from leukemia and other cancers among patients with Down's syndrome (mongols) and among their parents. *Br J Cancer.* 1962;16:177-186.

323.Jackson EW, Turner JH, Klauber MR, Norris FD. Down's syndrome: variation of leukemia occurrence in institutionalized populations. *J Chron Dis.* 1968;21:247-253.

324.Wald N, Borges WH, Li CC, Turner JH, Harnois CD. Leukemia associated with mongolism. *Lancet.* 1961;1:1228.

325.Robison LL, Nesbit ME, Sather HN, Level C, Shahidi N, Kennedy A, Hammond D. Down syndrome and acute leukemia in children: a 10-year retrospective survey from Childrens Cancer Study Group. *J Pediatr.* 1984;105:235-242.

326.Kalwinsky DK, Ralmondi SC, Bunin NJ, Fairclough D, Pui CH, Relling MV, et al. Clinical and biological characteristics of acute lymphocytic leukemia in children with Down syndrome. *Am J Med Genet Suppl.* 1990;7:267-271.

327.Levitt GA, Stiller CA, Chessells JM. Prognosis of Down's syndrome with acute leukemia. *Arch Dis Child.* 1990;65:212-216.

328.Franceschi M, Comola M, Piattoni F, Gualandri W, Canal N. Prevalence of dementia in adult patients with trisomy 21. *Am J Med Genet Suppl.* 1990;7:306-308.

329.Evenhuis HM. The natural history of dementia in Down's syndrome. *Arch Neurol.* 1990;47:263-267.

330.Lai F, Williams RS. A prospective study of Alzheimer disease in Down syndrome. *Arch Neurol.* 1989;46:849-853.

331.Zigman WB, Schupf N, Lubin RA, Silverman WP. Premature regression of adults with Down syndrome. *Am J Ment Defic.* 1987;92:161-168.

332.Ball MJ, Nuttall K. Neurofibrillary tangles, granulovascular degeneration, and neuron loss in Down syndrome: quantitative comparison with Alzheimer dementia. *Ann Neurol.* 1980;7:462-465.

333.Ropper AH, Williams RS. Relationship between plaques, tangles, and dementia in Down syndrome. *Neurology.* 1980;30:639-644.

334.Blusztajn JK, Gonzales-Coviella IL, Logue M, Growdon JH, Wurtman RJ. Levels of phospholipid catabolic intermediates, glycerophosphocholine and glycerophosphoethanolamine, are elevated in brains of Alzheimer's disease but not of Down's syndrome patients. *Brain Res.* 1990;536:240-244.

335.Nelson KB. What proportion of cerebral palsy is related to birth asphyxia? *J Pediatr.* 1987;112:572-573.

336.Wollack JB, Low NL, Carter S. Static encephalopathies. In: Rudolph AM, Hoffman JIE, Randolph CD, eds. *Rudolph's Pediatrics.* Norwalk, Connecticut: Appleton Lange; 1991:1720-1724.

337.Nelson KB. Relationship of intrapartum and delivery room events to long-term neurologic outcome. *Clin Perinatol.* 1989;16:995-1007.

244 The Cost of Birth Defects

338.Nelson KB, Ellenberg JH. Antecedents of cerebral palsy: multivariate analysis of risk. *New Engl J Med.* 1986;315:81-86.

339.Torfs CP, van den Berg B, Oechsli FW, Cummins S. Prenatal and perinatal factors in the etiology of cerebral palsy. *J Pediatr.* 1990;116:615-619.

340.Blair E, Stanley FJ. Intrapartum asphyxia: a rare cause of cerebral palsy. *J Pediatr.* 1988;112:515-519.

341.Rantakallio P, Von Wendt L. A prospective comparative study of the aetiology of cerebral palsy and epilepsy in a one-year birth cohort from northern Finland. *Acta Pediatr Scand.* 1986;75:586-592.

342.Wright R, Nicholson J. Physiotherapy for the spastic child: an evaluation. *Dev Med Child Neurol.* 1973;15:146-163.

343.Pharoah POD, Cooke T, Cooke RWI, Rosenbloom L. Birthweight specific trends in cerebral palsy. *Arch Dis Child.* 1990;65:602-606.

344.Stanley FJ, Watson L. The cerebral palsies in Western Australia: trends, 1968 to 1981. *Am J Obstet Gynecol.* 1988;158:89-93.

345.Emond A, Golding J, Peckham C. Cerebral palsy in two national cohort studies. *Arch Dis Child.* 1989;64:848-852.

346.Veall RM. Ibid.

347.Ingram TTS. A study of cerebral palsy in the childhood population of Edinburgh. *Arch Dis Child.* 1955;30:85-98.

348.Asher P, Schonell FE. A survey of 400 cases of cerebral palsy in childhood. *Arch Dis Child.* 1950;25:360-379.

349.Wendt L, Rantakallio P, Saukkonen AL, Tuisku M, Makinen H. Cerebral palsy and additional handicaps in a 1-year birth cohort from Northern Finland: a prospective follow-up study to the age of 14 years. *Ann Clin Res.* 1985;17:156-161.

350.Kudrjavcev T, Schoenberg BS, Kurland LT, Groover RV. Cerebral palsy: survival rates, associated handicaps, and distribution by clinical subtype (Rochester, MN, 1950-1976). *Neurol.* 1985;35:900-903.

351.Perlstein MA, Hood PN. Infantile spastic hemiplegia. III. intelligence. *Pediatrics.* 1955;15:676-682.

352.Uvebrant P. Hemiplegic cerebral palsy: aetiology and outcome. *Acta Paediatr Scand Suppl.* 1988;345:1-100.

353.Edebol-Tysk K. Epidemiology of spastic tetraplegic cerebral palsy in Sweden. I. impairments and disabilities. *Neuropediatr.* 1989;20:41-45.

354.Abbott R, Forem SL, Johann M. Selective posterior rhizotomy for the treatment of spasticity: a review. *Child Nerv System.* 1989;5:337-346.

355.Klapper ZS, Birch HG. The relation of childhood characteristics to outcome in young adults with cerebral palsy. *Develop Med Child Neurol.* 1966;8:645-656.

356.Veall RM. Ibid.

357.Abbott R, et al. Ibid.

358.Robinson RO. The frequency of other handicaps in children with cerebral palsy. *Develop Med Child Neurol.* 1973;15:305-312.

359.Evans P, Elliott M, Alberman E, Evans S. Prevalence and disabilities in 4 to 8 year olds with cerebral palsy. *Arch Dis Child.* 1985;60:940-945.

360.Bhat M, Nelson KB. Developmental enamel defects in primary teeth in children with cerebral palsy, mental retardation, or hearing defects: a review. *Adv Dent Res.* 1989;3(2):132-142.

361.Thometz JG, Simon SR. Progression of scoliosis after skeletal maturity in institutionalized adults who have cerebral palsy. *J Bone Joint Surg.* 1988;70-A:1290-1296.

362.Harris SR, Atwater SW, Crowe TK. Accepted and controversial neuromotor therapies for infants at high risk for cerebral palsy. *J Perinatol.* 1988;8:3-13.

363.Palmer FB, Shapiro BK, Wachtel RC, Allen MC, Hiller JE, Harryman SE, et al. The effects of physical therapy on cerebral palsy: a controlled trial in infants with spastic diplegia. *New Engl J Med.* 1988;318:803-808.

364.Wright R, Nicholson J. Ibid.

365.Scherzer AL, Mike V, Ilson J. Physical therapy as a determinant of change in the cerebral palsied infant. *Pediatrics.* 1976;58:47-52.

366.Goodman M, Rothberg AD, Houston-McMillan JE, et al. Effect of early neurodevelopmental therapy in normal and at-risk survivors of neonatal intensive care. *Lancet.* 1985;2:1327-1331.

367.Piper MC, Kunos I, Willis DM, et al. Early physical therapy effects on the high-risk infant: a randomized controlled trial. *Pediatrics.* 1986;78:216-224.

368.Hanson CJ, Jones LJ. Gait abnormalities and inhibitive casts in cerebral palsy: literature review. *J Am Podiatr Med Assoc.* 1989;79(2):53-59.

369.Rosenthal RK. The use of orthotics in foot and ankle problems in cerebral palsy. *Foot Ankle.* 1984;4:195.

370.Milla JJ, Jackson ADM. A controlled trial of baclofen in children with cerebral palsy. *J Int Med Res.* 1973;5:398.

371.Ford F, Bleck EE, Aptekam RG, et al. Efficacy of dantrolene sodium in the treatment of spastic cerebral palsy. *Dev Med Child Neurol.* 1976;18:770.

372.Thometz JG, Tachdjian M. Long-term follow-up of the flexor carpi ulnaris transfer in spastic hemiplegic children. *J Pediatr Orthop.* 1988;8:407-412.

373.Peterson HA, Coventry MB. Long-term results of surgical treatment of adults with cerebral palsy. *Develop Med Child Neurol.* 1969;11:35-43.

374.Spencer JD. Mobility of the young adult physically handicapped patient following lower limb surgery in childhood. *J Royal Soc Med.* 1990;83:168-171.

375.Peacock WJ, Staudt LA. Spasticity in cerebral palsy and the selective posterior rhizotomy procedure. *J Child Neurol.* 1990;5:179-185.

376.Arens LJ, Peacock WJ, Peter J. Selective posterior rhizotomy: a long-term follow-up study. *Child Nerv System.* 1989;5:148-152.

377.Abbott R, et al. Ibid.

378.Landau WM, Hunt CC. Dorsal rhizotomy, a treatment of unproven efficacy (editorial). *J Child Neurol.* 1990;5:174-178.

379.Nelson KB, Ellenberg JH. Children who "outgrew" cerebral palsy. *Pediatrics.* 1982;69:529-536.

380.Taudorf K, Hansen FJ, Melchior JC, Pedersen H. Spontaneous remission of cerebral palsy. *Neuropediatr.* 1986;17:19-22.

381.Hutton JL, Cooke T, Pharoah POD. Life expectancy in children with cerebral palsy. *BMJ.* 1994;309:431-435.

382.Cohen P, Kohn JG. Follow-up study of patients with cerebral palsy. *West J Med.* 1979;130:6-11.

383.Andrews G, Platt LJ, Quinn PT, Neilson PD. An assessment of the status of adults with cerebral palsy. *Develop Med Child Neurol.* 1977;19:803-810.

384.O'Grady RS, Nishimura DM, Kohn JG, Bruvold WH. Vocational predictions compared with present vocational status of 60 young adults with cerebral palsy. *Develop Med Child Neurol.* 1985;27:775-784.

385.Magill J, Hurlbut N. The self-esteem of adolescents with cerebral palsy. *Am J Occup Med.* 1986;40:402-407.

386.Hutton JL, et al. Ibid.

Appendix 2

Description of Major Data Sources

This appendix provides a brief description of the eleven major data sources used for our cost estimates.

California Birth Defects Monitoring Program Incidence Data (CBDMP1)

The CBDMP is the largest active surveillance program for congenital anomalies in the world. The ascertainment area of the registry has expanded progressively since 1983 to encompass the entire state in 1990. The program, within the California Department of Health, employs data collection specialists who routinely visit hospitals and genetic centers where they review facility logs, identify all children up to one year of age diagnosed with reportable conditions, and record those conditions using British Pediatric Association codes.[1]

California Birth Defects Monitoring Program Linked Birth Death Records (CBDMP2)

The CBDMP conducted a special study merging the above CBDMP1 registry information from 1983-1986 with data from the

National Center for Health Statistic's linked birth-death file for California. The linked file merges death records with birth certificate information for all persons born in California who died in the first year of life.

National Health Interview Surveys, 1985-1989 (NHIS)

The NHIS is an annual survey conducted by the National Center for Health Statistics (NCHS) to assess the prevalence of chronic conditions, activity limitations due to health, and health care utilization in the United States general population. Each survey is a nationally representative sample containing records on approximately 100,000 individuals. The pooled five-year sample, therefore, contained approximately one-half million records. The estimated prevalence of any particular chronic condition from NHIS is based on the one-sixth sample of respondents presented with the one of six condition checklists on which the condition appears. NCHS has constructed "Recode C" categories aggregating one or several ICD-9 four-digit disease categories; thus, reliable national prevalence estimates of conditions can be made from a single survey.

California Office of Statewide Health Planning and Development Hospital Discharge Abstracts, 1988 (OSHPD)

The OSHPD data file contains hospital discharge abstracts from all acute-care, nonfederal hospitals in California for patients discharged in 1988. For each hospital discharge, the abstract contains the principal diagnosis (ICD-9-CM code) and up to twenty-four secondary diagnoses, as well as information on surgical procedures performed, length of stay, charges, expected source of payment, disposition at time of discharge, and demographic information such as age and sex. We used the subsample of OSHPD records that included a birth defect of interest in any primary or secondary diagnosis field.[a]

MediCal "Tape-to-Tape" Claims File, 1988 (MediCal)

The MediCal file is comprised of separate component files for inpatient, outpatient, and long-term care claims reimbursed by MediCal. In addition to other information, each claim record contains the MediCal recipient identification number, the principal diagnosis (ICD-9 code), charges, and the amount that MediCal paid. An additional "early returns" file provides summary data, by recipient identification number, on all claims by service type for the year as well as information on each recipient' s age, sex, and duration of MediCal eligibility. The MediCal subfile that we acquired contained all inpatient, outpatient, and long-term care claims for all MediCal recipients in 1988 who had at least one claim during the year with a diagnosis of interest recorded.

California Department of Developmental Services (DDS) Masterfile, 1988-1989 (DDS File)

The DDS file contains diagnostic, evaluative, and residential status data from the California Development and Evaluation Report (CDER) merged, by client identification number, with accounting data on purchases of developmental services for the fiscal year. In addition to listing the one or more of five qualifying conditions (mental retardation, cerebral palsy or like dysfunction, epilepsy, autism, or other condition similar or requiring services similar to mental retardation) for DDS services for each client, the CDER record contains, beginning in 1984, information on up to two underlying etiologies (ICD-9 codes) for each qualifying condition. Up to five additional medical conditions that contribute significantly to the developmental needs of the client also may be recorded (using ICD-9). The 10% random sample of this file (obtained from DDS)

---

[a]Additional surgical procedure codes were stipulated in extracting hospital discharge data for those with omphalocele.

contained approximately 9,000 records. Selection of the subsample, with birth defects of interest from the file, was based on anyone listed as having cerebral palsy as a qualifying condition for DDS services.[b] In addition to cerebral palsy, sufficient numbers of clients were found in the DDS file with Down syndrome, spina bifida, and cleft lip or palate (through age four) to generate reliable estimates of costs of developmental services for these conditions.

The National Longitudinal Transition Study of Special Education Students, 1990 (SRI)

This survey, conducted by Stanford Research International (SRI) in 1985, contains data on a nationally representative sample of approximately 8,500 secondary school special education students. The file contains separate parent, school record, and school district components, in addition to others, that can be linked by a respondent's identification number. Up to fourteen underlying disabilities/conditions from the parent questionnaire and up to seventeen such conditions from the school record abstract are provided in the file. The federal handicap category for each respondent (one of eleven) is assigned in the file based on an algorithm developed by SRI that utilizes information on placement from the school district or information on underlying disabilities in which district information was absent or otherwise inadequate.

California Special Education Enrollment Data, 1988-1989 (SPEED)

This file contains California special education enrollment data for the 1988-1989 school year by school district, age, federal handicap category, and placement category (designated instructional services,

---

[b]In 1986, the definition of cerebral palsy as a qualifying condition was expanded to include "like dysfunction." Based upon the observed 2% increase in the proportion of all DDS clients with cerebral palsy or like dysfunction after this change, we adjusted the expanded number downward to estimate the number of persons with cerebral palsy.

resource specialist, special day class, and nonpublic school) from the California Department of Education.

California Special Education Expenditure Data (SPEND), 1988-1989

This file contains district-level expenditures for special education by placement setting from the School Business Services Division of the California State Department of Education for all school districts in California in the 1988-1989 school year. These cost data include direct costs, direct support costs, and indirect costs as defined by the Department of Education.

Survey of Income and Program Participation, 1987, Wave 2 (SIPP)

SIPP is a cohort or "panel" survey conducted annually by the US Bureau of the Census on labor force participation, earnings and other income, assets, and receipt of support through various public programs. Each panel covers a nationally representative sample of approximately 30,000 households that are reinterviewed at five-month intervals for approximately two and a half years regarding the previous four months. Each interview is called a "Wave." Several waves contain "topical modules" on special issues of interest. Wave 2 of the 1987 panel contained a topical module on work disability among those ages sixteen to sixty-seven. In addition to listing general conditions such as mental retardation underlay such disabilities, SIPP collects data on the timing of and circumstances leading to the disability.

California Age-Sex Earnings Profiles, 1988

These lifetime earnings profiles incorporate age- and sex-specific labor market participation rates in 1989 from the US Department of Labor, life expectancy in 1989 from the California Department of

Health Services, and national earnings data from the US Bureau of the Census adjusted to California based upon aggregate earnings in the state relative to the nation. In addition to labor market earnings, these data include age- and sex-specific imputed values of household production. All of these data are adopted from the "under age one" detailed tables constructed by Rice and Max.[2] A 1% annual growth in actual productivity is assumed, and integrated into the figures. The figures are adjusted to 1988 based on the change in nominal compensation in the business sector in the United States between 1988 and 1989.

Endnotes to Appendix 2

1.Croen L, Schulman J, Roeper P. *Birth Defects in California: January 1, 1983-December 31, 1986.* Emeryville, California: California Birth Defects Monitoring Program; 1990.

2.Rice DP, Max W. *The Cost of Smoking in California, 1989.* Sacramento, California: California State Department of Health Services.

Index